Pediatric Assessment

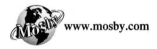www.mosby.com

POCKET GUIDE TO

Pediatric Assessment

Joyce Engel, RN, MEd, PhD(c)
Dean of Health Studies
Medicine Hat College
Medicine Hat, Alberta, Canada

Fourth Edition

with 85 illustrations

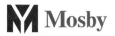 Mosby

An Imprint of Elsevier Science

St. Louis   London   Philadelphia   Sydney   Toronto

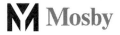

An Imprint of Elsevier Science

Vice President and Publishing Director, Nursing: Sally Schrefer
Senior Editor: Loren S. Wilson
Senior Developmental Editor: Michele D. Hayden
Publishing Services Manager: Catherine Jackson
Project Manager: Clay Broeker
Designer: Amy Buxton
Cover Photograph: Getty Images

Mosby, Inc.
An Imprint of Elsevier Science
11830 Westline Industrial Drive
St. Louis, Missouri 63146

Printed in the United States of America

Library of Congress Cataloging-in-Publication Data

Engel, Joyce.
    Pocket guide to pediatric assessment / Joyce Engel.—4th ed.
        p. ; cm.
    Includes bibliographical references and index.
    ISBN 0-323-01600-6
    1. Children—Medical examinations—Handbooks, manuals, etc. 2. Children—Diseases—Handbooks, manuals, etc. 3. Physical diagnosis—Handbooks, manuals, etc. 4. Pediatric nursing—Handbooks, manuals, etc.
    I. Title: Pediatric assessment. II. Title.
        [DNLM: 1. Pediatric Nursing—Handbooks. 2. Nursing Assessment—Child—Handbooks. 3. Physical Examination—Child—Handbooks.
    WY 49 E57p 2002]
    RJ50 .E64 2002
    618.92'0075—dc21   2001056246

02 03 04 05 06 GW/FF 9 8 7 6 5 4 3 2 1

Consultants

BARBARA W. BERG, RN, PNP, MN
Head Nurse,
Rose Children's Center at Rose Medical Center,
Denver, Colorado

DENA K. CUYJET, RN, MS, CPNP
Pediatric Nurse Practitioner,
Newborn Discharge Coordinator,
Kaiser Permanente San Francisco,
San Francisco, California

SHERRY D. FERKI, RN, MSN
Nurse Educator,
Louise Obici School of Nursing,
Suffolk, Virginia

TERRY FUGATE, RN, BSN
Formerly Adjunct and Associate Faculty,
Texas Tech University,
Health Sciences Center,
Lubbock, Texas

SARAH G. FULLER, RN, CPNP, PhD
Associate Professor,
College of Nursing,
University of South Carolina,
Columbia, South Carolina

SANDRA L. GARDNER, RN, MS, PNP
Director,
Professional Outreach Consultation,
Aurora, Colorado

MARILYN B. HARTSELL, RN, MSN
Coordinator,
Tri-Regional Education and Networking Development System,
University of Delaware,
Newark, Delaware

KAREN HALVORSON, RN, MN
Assistant Director of Nursing,
Manhattan Convalescent Home,
Tampa, Florida

CHRISTINA BERGH JACKSON, RN, CPNP, MSN
Pediatric Nurse Practitioner,
Pennsylvania School of the Deaf,
Philadelphia, Pennsylvania;
Instructor,
Eastern College,
St. Davids, Pennsylvania

CAROL A. KILMON, RN, CPNP, MSN, PhD
Assistant Professor,
The University of Texas Medical Branch,
Galveston, Texas

CATHERINE F. NOONAN, RN, MS, CPNP
Nurse Practitioner,
Children's Hospital;
Assistant Professor,
Nurse Education Department,
Bunker Hill Community College,
Boston, Massachusetts

MARY ANN NORTON, RNC, CPNP, PhD
Associate Professor,
North Michigan University,
Marquette, Michigan

MARGARET C. SLOTA, RN, MN
Pediatrics Consultant,
Pittsburgh, Pennsylvania

JANET F. SULLIVAN, RN, C, PhD
Clinical Associate Professor,
Parent Child Health Nursing,
State of New York Health Sciences Center,
Stony Brook, New York

Preface

As in the previous editions, *Pocket Guide to Pediatric Assessment* seeks to provide student nurses and experienced nurses alike with accessible, current, and comprehensive information in a direct, practical, and concise format.

Organization and Approach

This edition continues to approach the health assessment of pediatric clients systematically, using body systems as a primary framework. The presentation of communication strategies, family assessment, home assessment, developmental assessment, and assessment of abuse provide broader contexts and strategies for assessment and guide the nurse to a holistic approach to children and families. Most sections are preceded with a discussion of developmental variations that are fundamental to the assessment approaches, techniques, and findings, and assist in rooting the assessment within the context of the pediatric client and family. Clinical alerts draw attention to significant findings and deviations from normal, and nursing diagnoses complete the process of assessment.

The New Edition

The new edition has been extensively revised to reflect trends in pediatric nursing, up-to-date techniques, and currency in findings. Expanded and new assessment material related to headaches and coughs has been organized into charts and complements the section on abdominal pain that was introduced in the last edition. Content and strategies pertinent to assessment of mental status, athletic injuries, nutrition, vital sign measurement, and substance abuse have been expanded, and updated growth charts and immunization schedules have been included to provide the basis for comprehensive, holistic, and practical assessment of infants, children, and adolescents.

Journeys

I am continuously reminded by our five children about the complexity, challenges, and constant evolution in the area of child health. Within the complexities of child health, we often need the wisdom of practical, concise guidelines to assist in making sound child- and family-centered decisions. It is my hope that this fourth edition of *Pocket Guide to Pediatric Assessment* will contribute the kind of practical, practice-based guidance that assists children and families toward positive coping in illness and toward embracing behaviors consistent with health.

Joyce Engel

Contents

Unit III   Assessment of Body Systems

HEALTH
HISTORY

I

Beginning the Assessment

The focus of this text is on health assessment of the child, beginning with the 1-month-old infant and ending with the teenager in late adolescence. Although the physical assessment process is broken down into evaluations of the various body systems, the nurse need not adopt a fragmented approach to physical assessment. In fact, physical assessment is continuous and occurs during the health interview, when the nurse is also able to observe the infant, child, or adolescent.

Assessment is facilitated for child, parent (if present), and examiner if a rapport is established early. It may not be possible to erase all of a child's apprehension or discomfort, but setting up a relationship of trust and communication can help make the assessment a more positive experience.

Guidelines for Communicating with Children

- Take time to become acquainted with the child and parents.
- Set up a physical environment that is appropriately warm, cheerful, and private. If possible, select an environment that is decorated in an age-appropriate manner; adolescents, for example, may not appreciate Snow White pictures.
- Ask the parents how the child usually copes with new or stressful situations or what previous experiences the child has had with health care or caregivers. Knowing how the child might react enables the nurse to plan specific interventions to facilitate communication.
- Ask the parents what they have told the child about the health care encounter. The preparation children receive, especially males, is often inadequate or inappropriate. If so, more time may be needed to prepare the child before beginning any aspect of the health assessment requiring active participation.

- Observe the child's behavior for clues to readiness. A child who is ready to participate in assessment will ask questions, make eye contact, describe past experiences, touch equipment, or detach willingly from the parent.
- Consider the child's developmental level and attention span and use an imaginative approach when planning the examination.
- If a child is having difficulty accepting the assessment:

   Talk to the parent, ignoring the child.
   Compliment the child.
   Play a game (such as peek-a-boo) or tell a story.
   Use the third-person linguistic form: "Sometimes a guy can get really scared when his blood pressure is taken."
   Sequence the assessment from the least discomfort to the most discomfort.
   Start from toe to head.
   Undress the child gradually or allow the child to undress gradually.
   Briefly perform the technique on the parent first.

- Encourage the child to ask questions during assessment, but do not pressure to do so. This allows the child some control over the situation.
- Explain the assessment process in terms consistent with the child's developmental level.
- Use concrete terms rather than technical information, particularly with younger children: "I can hear you breathing in and out," not "I am auscultating your chest." "Do your ears ever hurt?" not "Have you had otitis media?"
- Present small amounts of information at a time. A rule of thumb is that no more than three items should be presented at once.
- Do not make rushed movements.
- Make expectations known clearly and simply: "I want you to be very still."
- *Do not offer choice where there is none.*
- Offer honest praise: "I know that hurt. You held your tummy very still." A positive experience helps build coping skills and self-esteem.
- If using an interpreter, it is critical to explain the purpose of the assessment and to introduce the interpreter to the family. Avoid medical jargon as much as possible, and ask one question at a time.

■ When examining more than one child, usually begin with the oldest or most cooperative child.

Communicating with Infants

Infants (1 to 12 months) primarily communicate through nonverbal vocalization and crying and respond to nonverbal communication behaviors of adults, such as holding, rocking, and patting. It is useful to observe the parent's or significant other's interpretation of the infant's nonverbal cues and the nonverbal communications of the parents. These established communication patterns can aid the nurse in setting up rapport with the infant.

Young infants respond well to gentle physical contact with any adult, but older infants may evidence strong separation and stranger anxieties. If it is necessary to handle the older infant, do so firmly while avoiding abrupt movements and preparatory gestures such as holding out hands or coaxing the child to come. Although infants younger than 6 months usually tolerate lying on the examining table, older infants and toddlers are more comfortable when held or sitting in the parent's or caregiver's lap. As much as possible, carry out the assessment in a way that allows the infant to either keep the parent in view or to be held by the parent. Infants should be allowed security objects such as blankets and pacifiers, if they have them. The use of a high-pitched, soft voice and smile will also assist in gaining the infant's cooperation.

Communicating with Toddlers

Toddlers (12 months to 3 years) have not yet acquired the ability to effectively communicate verbally. Their communication is rich with expressive nonverbal gestures and simple verbal communications. Pushing the examiner's hand away and crying can be an eloquent expression of fear, anxiety, or lack of knowledge. Toddlers accept the verbal communications of others literally, so that saying, "I can see all the way to your tummy button when you open your mouth" will mean just that to toddlers. Toddlers have the beginnings of memory and make believe, but they are unable to understand abstractions and become frustrated and frightened by phrases that seem ordinary to adults. Perceptions of threat are amplified by inaccurate understandings of the situation and limited knowledge of the resources that are available.

Communication with toddlers requires that the nurse use short, concrete terms. Explanations and descriptions need to be repeated several times. Visual aids such as puppets and dolls assist explanations. Children of this age attribute magical qualities to inanimate objects, so it is useful to allow them to handle instruments and to tell them exactly, in concrete terms, what the instrument does and how it feels. The use of comfort objects and access to the parent should be encouraged throughout the assessment, as they are for the infant.

Communicating with Preschool-Aged Children

Although preschoolers (3 to 6 years) generally use more sophisticated verbal communications, their reasoning is intuitive. Therefore many of the guidelines for communicating with toddlers apply to preschoolers as well. Because of the preschooler's increased verbal communication abilities, the nurse can successfully indicate to the child how and when cooperation is desired. The older preschooler, in particular, likes to conform, knows most external body parts, and may be interested in the purpose of various parts of the assessment. Allowing the preschooler to handle the equipment eases fears and helps answer questions about how the equipment is used.

Preschool-aged children are often very modest. They should be exposed minimally during examination and requested to undress themselves. They need to know exactly what is being examined and benefit from opportunities for questions. Parental proximity is still important for this age-group.

Communicating with School-Aged Children

School-aged children (6 to 12 years) think in concrete terms but at a more sophisticated level. Generally they have had enough contact with health care personnel that they can rely on past experiences to guide them. Depending on the quality of their past experiences, they may appear shy or reticent during health assessment. Frequently they may fear injury or embarrassment. Allowing time for composure and privacy (perhaps even from parents) aids in communication. Reassurance and third-person speech are helpful in eliciting fears and anxieties and in allowing the child to express hurt.

The purpose of the health assessment should be related to the child's condition. It is useful to determine what the child already knows about the health contact and to proceed from there. Simple medical diagrams and teaching dolls are useful in explaining the assessment process. Specific information should be given about body parts affected by the assessment.

Children of this age are often curious about the function of equipment and its usefulness. An appropriate response to "How can you tell what my temperature is from the thermometer?" might be "Your body heat pushes the silver up the glass tube. I can then read how far the silver has been pushed up the scale on the tube."

Communicating with Adolescents

Adolescents (12 years and older) use sophisticated verbal communication, although their behavior may not necessarily indicate an advanced level of communication, cognition, or maturity. Adolescents may respond to verbal approaches with monosyllables, reticence, anger, or other behaviors, and the nurse may have to do more talking than is usual at the beginning of the interaction. The nurse must avoid the tendency to respond to less than desirable social behaviors with prying, confrontation, continuous questioning, or judgmental attitudes. Easing into the initial contact with discussion of friends, hobbies, school, and family can give the apprehensive adolescent time for self-composure. Disclosure may occur more easily when the adolescent and nurse are engaged in joint activity.

It is helpful to ask the adolescent what he or she knows about the health contact and to explain the rationale for the health assessment. Adolescents may be concerned about privacy and confidentiality, and opportunity should be provided for completing some or all of the assessment without the presence of the parent. The female nurse needs to be sensitive to the potential of embarrassment for male adolescents at being examined by a female and provide draping and minimal touching. The parameters of confidentiality should be explained; specifically, it should be explained that disclosure is confidential unless intervention is necessary. Adolescents tend to be preoccupied with body image and function, and when appropriate they should be given feedback from the assessment. Diagrams and models can enhance feedback. Although adolescents have a high level of comprehension and vocabulary, they may not consistently function at higher levels of cognition, and the nurse must avoid the tendency to become too abstract, too detailed, and too technical. The self-conscious adolescent may be reluctant to ask for clarification of an explanation that has not been understood.

Communicating with Parents

Parents are often an integral part of the health assessment of an infant or child. Parents are the primary source of information about the young child. The information that parents give can be considered reliable in most instances because of close contact with their children.

Broad questions are useful, especially in eliciting responses in sensitive areas, because the parent can assume control over the direction of the response: "Tell me what Jason did at 2 years" is less threatening than "Did Jason talk when he was 2?" or "Did you have trouble disciplining Jason when he was 2?" More focused and closed questions should be saved for later in the assessment process when specific information is desired.

The use of silence and of listening is essential in reassuring parents that what they are about to say is worthwhile. In a supportive, attentive atmosphere, parents often communicate information and feelings that may have little to do with the current problem but have great significance in the overall care of the child.

The parents are members of the health team. If they believe the child has a problem, their concern must be treated seriously. The parents and the nurse must agree that the problem exists. Once agreement exists, the nurse can ask how the parents have tried to solve the problem. This approach reinforces the worth of the parents' solutions. Having accomplished this, the nurse can help the parents to find alternative solutions for the problem. Occasionally parents will select alternatives that are not preferred. If the alternative will not harm the child, it is best to allow the parents to carry out their plan.

The nurse must avoid the temptation to inundate the parents with anticipatory guidance. Parents need recognition, praise, and reassurance for their strengths. Too much information and advice can intimidate parents and effectively shut down communication.

Communicating with Parents and Children from Diverse Cultures

In communicating with parents and children from diverse cultures, it is critical to appreciate that communication patterns, childrearing practices, and health practices may differ from those of the nurse (Table 1-1). Knowledge of these differences will assist in developing hypotheses about the family and in acquiring sensitivity to differences; however, the nurse must observe the family carefully for cues to family practices and relationships with children and each other. Further, the nurse must avoid the trap of assuming that because the family belongs to a specific ethnic or cultural group, they will behave and hold beliefs similar to those of the group as a whole.

Establishing a Setting for the Health History

The health interview provides an ideal opportunity to establish communication and rapport and usually is the first step in an assessment. The interview should be conducted in a room that is private, bright, and nonthreatening. Toys and drawing materials are useful for distracting the young child, so that the parent can give the interviewer fuller attention.

Before beginning the health interview, nurses must introduce themselves and ask the names of family members. Family members are then addressed by name. Unless an infant, the child is usually included in the interview; the extent of involvement varies with age and culture.

Nurses must clarify their roles in the assessment process because in some health settings many health practitioners see the child. The purposes of the health interview and physical assessment are clarified because parents may wonder about the relevance of the information they are about to give. Parents, and the child, as appropriate, are also told who has access to the information and are assured about the limits of access. Once the parameters of the interview and physical assessment have been set, the parents are better able to decide how and what they wish to communicate.

Table 1-1 Cultural Variations in Family and Health Practices

	Family Structure	Child-Rearing	Traditional Health Care Beliefs/Practices	Relationship with Professionals	Prevalent Health Concerns
Cambodians/ Laotians	• Family key social and economic unit. • Extended family source of support and assistance. • Husband is head of household, decision maker. • Family problems are considered private.	• Physical discipline rare; discipline occurs through verbal admonition. • Respect for older siblings, adults predominant. • Children learn through observation and imitation. • Infants carried a great deal; not allowed to cry, walk later than Western children.	• Coin rubbing, using a coin or metal spoon, is used to treat a variety of common ailments. • Pinching involves pinching area between eyebrows until it turns red. Pinching and coin rubbing may leave bruising. • Ginseng, Tiger Balm are common self-treatments.	• Tend to seek professional help only if very ill. • Passive role in therapeutic relationship. • Expect treatments and medications. • May see blood tests as life threatening.	• Tuberculosis • Intestinal parasites • Anemia • Hepatitis B • Dental caries

Vietnamese	• Family main source of identity. • While traditional households often include grandparents, unmarried children, an adult couple, and children, traumatic circumstances have separated many from family members in Vietnam. May limit ability to become established in new surroundings. • Women have	• Most training is through example. • Discipline may include quiet verbal admonition, shouting, or slapping. • Beatings, although rare, are considered to be private family matters. • Quiet compliance is expected of children; open anger rare but children may express anger through stubbornness or passive noncooperation.	• Herbal remedies, isolation of sick, and visits to shrines practiced. • Ideas of health center around hereditary causes of illness, supernatural causes of illness, hot and cold equilibrium, and good and bad wind and water. • Being "hot" may refer to having a symptom believed caused by heat imbalance in body—	• Regard physicians very highly; public health nurses more highly regarded than other nurses because they are government employees. • Visits are expected to be formal, unhurried, without detailed questions about health or social background. • Touching and removal of clothing produces discomfort. • Stoical with	• Hepatitis B • Pulmonary tuberculosis • Intestinal parasites • Incomplete immunization • Constipation • Malnutrition • Anemia

Continued

Table 1-1 Cultural Variations in Family and Health Practices—cont'd

	Family Structure	Child-Rearing	Traditional Health Care Beliefs/Practices	Relationship with Professionals	Prevalent Health Concerns
Vietnamese —cont'd	fewer rights than men.		not necessarily fever. • Coin rubbing or placing a hot cup on the body may leave bruises.	illness and pain. • More accepting of prescription than of changes in their behavior.	
Chinese	• Large, extended families in a single household; unmarried children at home until marriage. • Husband is bread winner, takes care of finances, and	• Discipline may seem harsh to Westerners. • Open affection rarely displayed. • Toilet training initiated early. • High value placed on success in school and work.	• Practices based on a combination of folk, traditional, and modern medicine. • Word of mouth, family practices, magic, and religion important. • Illness results	• Health professionals highly respected; Chinese patient may not question out of respect. • May find team approach confusing as Chinese more familiar with	• Hepatitis • Tuberculosis • Intestinal parasites • Lactose intolerance • Dental caries

disciplines children. Wife takes care of household and usually makes health decisions. Divorce considered a disgrace.
- Serious decisions may involve **all** family members.
- Young obliged to take care of elderly.

from disequilibrium of opposing forces.
- Cures are sought from substances associated with perceived deficiencies (e.g., eating brains to get wiser).
- Food is essential to harmony with nature and is used to explain causes of illness and to treat disease.

having a close relationship with one or two professionals.
- Prefer older professionals and Chinese physicians if available.
- High expectations of treatment; may not understand limitations.
- Prevention difficult to understand because many Chinese seek help only when ill.

Continued

Table 1-1   Cultural Variations in Family and Health Practices—cont'd

	Family Structure	Child-Rearing	Traditional Health Care Beliefs/Practices	Relationship with Professionals	Prevalent Health Concerns
Hispanics	• Couple expected to set up independent household but has close ties with extended family. • Extended family includes blood relatives and godparents. • Husband is responsible for work outside the home and wife for household duties. • Physical force acceptable in arguments. • Men give orders	• More physical aggression present in urban than in rural families. • Children tend to play in groups and to roam neighborhood. • Children highly desired and valued. • Children may react strongly to separation from mother.	• Physicians are held in high esteem; nurses may not be highly esteemed. • Health professional needs to avoid going directly into health concerns; talk first about unrelated matters. • Prescriptions are expected. Careful explanations about alternative measures, diagnostic assessments,	• May associate hospitalization with death. • May resist bathing a fevered child. • Health is achieved through temperature equilibrium. Some medications, such as antibiotics, may be seen as "hot" and therefore as undesirable for a fever. • Disabled may be restricted	• Malnutrition • Dental caries • Scabies • Fevers • Bronchitis • Eczema • Worms • Parasites • Diabetes • Lead poisoning

Continued

to women and older give orders to younger. • Grandparents often involved in major decisions. • Family honor is important.	and preventive measures are beneficial. • May be late for appointments due to present time orientation. • Females will bring female relatives when visiting male professionals: Discussion of sexuality is taboo for a female in the presence of a male.	to privacy of home.	
Iranians	• Extended family considered important for advice, support, and for employment,	• Verbal abuse may be common; spanking is less common. • Children have	• Highly fatalistic; what occurs is the will of God. • Hot and cold used to treat minor illnesses.	• Older, male health professionals (especially physicians) generally preferred.

Table 1-1   Cultural Variations in Family and Health Practices—cont'd

	Family Structure	Child-Rearing	Traditional Health Care Beliefs/Practices	Relationship with Professionals	Prevalent Health Concerns
Iranians —cont'd	security, and influence. • Paternal influence strong. • Sex roles are very strong. • Children are least respected in family.	many limits. • Children have little say in family matters.	• Thin children are believed unhealthy; children tend to be overfed.	• Health visits need to allow time for undivided attention and to listen to long accounts of health and personal matters. • Personal relationship sought with caregiver. • Expect diagnostic tests and prescriptions. • Several family members may contact health professional about client.	

| South Asians | • Family most important social unit.
• Extended family tend to live in one household.
• Lifestyle collectivistic rather than individualistic.
• Earnings shared in the extended family.
• Head of household is the most established and financially secure male; head of household makes most decisions but consults close relatives | • Children relatively more controlled and protected than are North American children.
• Compliance achieved through threats, treats, and occasional spanking.
• Independence not encouraged.
• No fixed schedule for young children.
• Male children are preferred and have special roles.
• Education highly valued. | • Illnesses result from imbalance in body humors (bile, wind, phlegm).
• Dietary imbalance most common cause of sickness.
• Bathing, massage, ritual oils, herbs, and foods are used to treat ailments. | • Physician expected to have all the answers, make all decisions, and go beyond questions.
• Medication is expected.
• Formal dress expected in caregivers.
• Females tend to be uncomfortable with male caregivers.
• Health care decisions about children made by senior family members.
• Care of ill family members | • Tuberculosis
• Parasites
• Hepatitis
• Malaria |

Continued

Table 1-1   Cultural Variations in Family and Health Practices—cont'd

	Family Structure	Child-Rearing	Traditional Health Care Beliefs/Practices	Relationship with Professionals	Prevalent Health Concerns
South Asians —cont'd	on matters of importance. • Wife is seen as husband's possession.			is responsibility of wife, grandparents.	
Native Americans	• Many variations in family structure and values. • Tribe and extended family tend to come before self. • Elders are source of wisdom. • Extended family structures.	• Children learn through observation, imitation, legends. • Male child held in higher esteem than female child.	• Health is a state of harmony with nature. • Spirituality interwoven with medicine. • All disorders believed to have element of supernatural. • Native healers used in some tribes. • Do not believe in germ theory.	• Going to hospital associated with illness. • Native American healers ask few questions. • Present, not future oriented, therefore preventive practices difficult to understand. • Time is on a continuum, therefore set	• Tuberculosis • Suicide • Lactose intolerance • Drug/alcohol abuse • Accidents

Blacks	• Strong kinship ties and interaction with extended family. • Kinship network not necessarily limited to blood lines; unrelated persons found in same household.	• High emphasis on peoplehood or collective consciousness. • Strong emphasis on ambition and work.	• Self-care, folk medicine important. • Tend to seek help from "old lady," priest, root doctor, spiritualist, or minister when ill.	• Illnesses prevented through religious rituals and charms.	intervals (such as with medication dosing) may need careful explanation. • Take time to form opinions of health professionals. • Silence, avoiding direct eye contact show respect. • Sensitive to any evidence of discrimination. • May disguise health concern initially to "test" health care professional's ability to see real problem.	• Sickle cell disease • Diabetes • Pneumonia • Cardiovascular disease • Lactose intolerance (preschoolers and older)

Continued

Table 1-1 Cultural Variations in Family and Health Practices—cont'd

	Family Structure	Child-Rearing	Traditional Health Care Beliefs/Practices	Relationship with Professionals	Prevalent Health Concerns
Blacks —cont'd	• Rigid sex roles deemphasized. • Men and women share in household and family responsibilities. • Turn to families, friends, neighbors, or minister in time of crisis. • Discussion of family concerns outside of family major breach of family ethics.		• Prayer important to healing and treatment. • Illness seen as "will of God." • May believe in voodoo and religious healing. • May wear copper and silver bracelets to prevent illness. • Prevention important through cleanliness, laxatives, rest, and diet.	• Nonverbal behavior important in interactions. • May deny need for help to avoid appearing helpless or dependent.	• Obesity • Drug/alcohol use

| Low income | • Relationships and behaviors influenced by social and economic stressors. | • Illness is inevitable.
• Health defined in terms of work; more important to work than to lose pay.
• Use self-care because of costs of health care.
• Death and dying inevitable due to poverty. | • May rely on emergency services for care.
• Relationships with caregivers may be short-lived.
• High infant mortality due to limited prenatal care and follow-up. | • Communicable diseases
• Infant mortality
• Drug/alcohol abuse
• Diabetes |

Dimensions of a History

2

Obtaining a health history is an important component of the health assessment process. The health interview assists in establishing rapport with the parent and child, provides data from which tentative nursing diagnoses can be made, offers an opportunity for the nurse and family to establish goals, and affords the opportunity for the nurse to provide education and support to the family.

The purposes and extent of the health interview varies with the nature of the health care contact. For example, in an emergency situation it is necessary to focus on the chief complaint and the details of past health care contacts. The prenatal and postnatal histories and the psychosocial dimensions can be left for later, unless they are the focus for the concern. When a child has repeated contacts with a health care facility, it is necessary only to update a health history if it has been completed on initial contact. The course of an interview must be modified to fit the situation and the setting. A home setting, for example, may include many distractions and will require adaptation to the family's environment.

Guidelines for Interviewing Parents and Children

- Follow principles of communication during the interview (see Chapter 1).
- Before beginning the interview the nurse must thoroughly understand the purposes of the health history and of the questions that are asked.
- If a specific illness or health concern is the reason for the interview, knowledge of the diagnosis helps focus questions related to the chief complaint. The nurse must also be alert to concerns raised by the parent or child that are not related to the diagnosis.
- Explain the purpose of the interview, before starting, to the parents and to the child. Cooperation and sharing are more likely

to occur if the parents understand that the questions facilitate better care for their child. For the adolescent, understanding the parameters of confidentiality may be crucial to what is shared.

■ Write brief notations about specific derails. *Do not try to write finished sentences,* and *keep writing to a minimum.* The flow of contact is lost if the nurse spends an extended amount of time writing or in staring at a form. Further, the nurse may miss important opportunities to observe behaviors and family inter- actions if overly committed to recording during the interview.

■ Know what information is necessary so that the parents and child are not asked for the same type of information repeatedly. *Repeat questions only if further clarification is desired.*

■ Give broad openings at the beginning of the interview, such as "Tell me why you came to see me today." Use direct questions, such as "Are the stools watery?" to assist the parent to focus on specific details.

■ Do not interrupt the parent, child, or parent and interpreter.

■ Accept what is being said. Nodding, reestablishing eye contact, or saying "uh-huh" provides encouragement to continue. If an interpreter is being used, avoid commenting about the family in the presence of the family.

■ Listen, and attend to nonverbal cues. The presenting complaint may have little to do with the real concern.

■ Convey empathy and an unhurried attitude. Sit at eye level, if possible. Observe the family from another culture to determine what behaviors are acceptable to them and, therefore, empathic to them. Eye contact, for example, is considered disrespectful in some cultures (e.g., Native Americans) rather than indicative of active listening and empathy.

■ Ensure mutual understanding. *Clarify* if unsure, and summarize for the parent and child what has been understood.

■ Integrate the child when possible and when culturally appropri- ate. Even the very young can answer the question "What do you like to eat?"

■ Be sensitive to the need to separately interview parents and child, particularly if the child is an adolescent.

■ Be sensitive to the need to consider who is responsible for health decisions in the family and for child care (see Chapter 1).

Information for Comprehensive History

Information	Comment
Date of History	Identifying Data
Include name, nickname, parents' (or guardians') names, home telephone number, number where parents (or guardians) can be reached during working hours, child's date of birth, age (months, years), sex, race, language spoken, language understood.	Much of this information may already be on a child's nameplate or chart.
Source of Referral, if Any	
Source of Information	
Include judgment about reliability of information.	
Chief Complaint	
Use broad opening statements, such as "What concerns bring you here today?" Record parents' or child's own words: "Running to the bathroom since Saturday."	Note who has identified the chief complaint. In some instances a schoolteacher or physician may have expressed the concern. Agreement between parents and another referral source is important to care. Adolescents and parents may differ regarding perception of complaint.
Present Illness	
Include a chronologic narrative of the chief complaint. The narrative answers questions related to *where* (location), *what* (quality, factors that aggravate or relieve symptoms), *when* (onset, duration, frequency), and *how much* (intensity, severity). The parent	Parents may need assistance in sorting out details. Prior knowledge of diagnosis aids in planning specific questions; however, care must be taken to avoid premature closure or diminished openness to possibilities not presented by the diagnosis. In a primary care

Information	Comment
or child should also be asked about associated manifestations. Include significant negatives: "The parent denies that the child has experienced undue fatigue, bruising, or joint tenderness." Inquire about what home and formal health care interventions have been tried to deal with the concern. Use direct questions to focus on specific details, as necessary.	setting, the nurse often begins by addressing health maintenance or health-promoting issues.

Information about previously tried home and health care interventions provide important data about parent/child knowledge of interventions, self-care abilities, motivation, and cultural practices. Some folk remedies can be harmful. For example, two folk remedies from Mexico that are used to treat colic contain lead (azarcon and greta).

Clinical Alert

Persistent denial in the face of unexplained or vaguely defined injuries may signal child abuse. Denial may also indicate nonacceptance of a concern such as a developmental delay or behavior problem.

Insistent presentation of symptoms (especially by mother) in the absence of objective data may be suggestive of Munchausen syndrome by proxy.

Past Medical History

General state of health

Inquire about appetite, recent weight losses or gains, fatigue, stresses.	Do not include information that may have been elicited for chief complaint or present illness.

Information	Comment
Birth history	
Include prenatal history (maternal health, infections, drugs taken [prescription and illegal]; tobacco and alcohol use; abnormal bleeding, weight gain, duration of pregnancy, attitudes toward pregnancy, birth, duration of labor, type of delivery, complications, birth weight, condition of infant at birth), and neonatal history (respiratory distress, cyanosis, jaundice, seizures, poor feeding, patterns of sleeping).	Birth history is especially important if the child is younger than 2 years or is experiencing developmental or neurologic problems.
Feeding	
For infants, include type of feeding (bottle, breast, solid foods), frequency of feedings, quantity of feeds, responses to feeding, types of foods, specific problems with feeding (colic, regurgitation, lethargy). For children, include self-feeding abilities, likes and dislikes, appetite, and amounts of food taken. For adolescents, include usual eating patterns and daily caloric intake.	Guidelines for a more complete nutritional history are supplied in Chapter 7. **Clinical Alert** Skipping meals may be the strongest predictor of inadequate calcium intake in adolescents.
Previous illnesses, operations, or injuries	
Include dates of hospitalizations, reasons for hospitalizations, and responses to illnesses.	Knowing how a child has reacted in past hospitalizations can help in planning interventions for a current hospitalization.

Information	Comment
Childhood illnesses	
Include the common communicable diseases, such as measles, mumps, and chickenpox. Inquire about recent contacts with persons with communicable diseases.	
Immunizations	
Include specific details about immunizations (dates, types) and untoward reactions. If a child has not been immunized, note the reason. Note desensitization procedures.	MMR vaccine contains chick embryo tissue that may trigger a reaction in egg-sensitive patients.
Current medications	
Include prescription and nonprescription drugs, dose, frequency, duration of use, time of last dose, and understanding of parents and/or child about the prescribed drugs.	
Allergies	
Include agent *and* reaction.	Knowing the reaction is useful because reactions may not be indicative of allergic manifestations.
Growth and Development	
Physical	
Include approximate height and weight at 1, 2, 5, and 10 years, and tooth eruption/loss.	A thorough history of growth and development is important in planning nursing interventions appropriate to the child's level and in screening for developmental and neurologic problems. A social history can identify the need for anticipatory guidance.
Developmental history	
Include ages at which child rolled over, sat alone, crawled, walked, spoke first words, spoke first sentences, and dressed without help.	

Information	Comment

Social history

Include toileting (age at which daytime and nighttime control were achieved or current level of control, enuresis, encopresis, self-toileting abilities, terminology used); sleep (amount and patterns during day and night, bedtime rituals and security objects, fears, and nightmares); speech (lisping, stuttering, intelligibility); sexuality (relationships with members of opposite sex, inquisitiveness about sexual information and activity, type of information given child); schooling (grade level in school, academic achievement, adjustment to school); habits (thumb sucking, nail biting, pica, head banging); discipline (methods used, child's response to discipline); and personality and temperament (congeniality, aggressiveness, temper tantrums, withdrawal, relationships with peers and family). Children and adolescents should be asked if they ever feel sad or "down." If yes, they should be asked if they have ever thought of killing themselves.

Behavior and temperament may provide important diagnostic and intervention information. Children with hearing impairments as well as school-aged children who experience recurrent abdominal pain are more likely to have difficult temperaments. Children with chronic cardiac disease are more intense, withdrawn, and more negative in mood than healthy children. Boys from violent home environments tend to bully, be argumentative, and have temper tantrums and short attention spans. Girls from violent homes tend to be anxious or depressed, to cling, and to be perfectionists. Infants born to mothers on cocaine exhibit sleep problems.

Behaviors, such as those related to toilet training, vary with culture. Open discussion of sexual matters may be restricted in some cultures (e.g., Hispanics).

Information	Comment

Family History

Include the ages and health of immediate family members, familial diseases, presence and types of congenital anomalies, consanguinity of parents, occupations and education of parents, and family interactions, including who is primarily responsible for childcare and for making decisions related to health care.

A genogram (Figure 2-1) is useful for showing the relationships, ages, health of family members, and who is in the household. (See Chapter 3 for a more detailed family assessment.) Needs of health care programs should be balanced with needs of families. Parents identify their main needs as information about diagnosis, effect of diagnosis on development, information about treatment, and effect of condition on sexuality of child.

Clinical Alert

Be alert to symptoms of lead poisoning in children whose siblings or playmates are being treated for lead poisoning.

Parental age of less than 18 years at the time of child's birth may be a risk factor for maltreatment.

Systems Review

1. General
2. Integument
3. Head and neck
4. Ears
5. Eyes
6. Face and nose
7. Thorax and lungs
8. Cardiovascular
9. Abdominal
10. Genitourinary/reproductive
11. Musculoskeletal
12. Neurologic

Questions appropriate for each system are included under the heading of "Preparation" in chapters of this book.

A

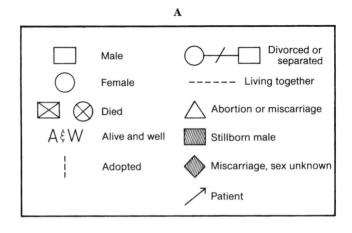

B

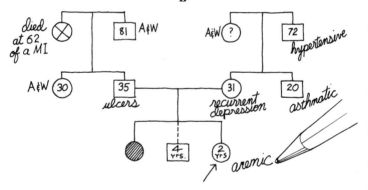

Figure 2-1

Constructing a genogram. **A,** Symbols used in a genogram.
B, Sample genogram.

Family Assessment

3

Assessment of the family includes exploration of structure, function, and developmental stage. Although family *therapy* is within the practice realm of those with special education and supervision, assessment is appropriate for practitioners with general preparation.

The assessment guidelines outlined in this chapter are adapted from those outlined by Wright and Leahey (1984) in the Calgary Family Assessment Model (CFAM) and reflect its strongly supported systems approach to family care.

Rationale

The family should be viewed as interacting, complex elements. The decisions and activities of one family member affect the others, and the family has an impact on the individual. Understanding family members' interactions and communications, family norms and expectations, how decisions are made, and how the family balances individual and family needs enables the nurse to understand the family's responses and needs during times of stress and well-being. This understanding can enrich the relationship between the nurse and family. The nurse's positive, proactive responses to family concerns and capabilities can help the family promote the development and well-being of its members.

General Concepts Related to Assessment

The primary premise in family systems assessment is that individuals are best understood in the context of their families. Studying a child and a parent as separate units does not constitute family assessment because it neglects observation of interactions. The parents and children are part of subsystems within a larger family system, which in turn is part of a larger subsystem.

Changes in any one of these systems components affect the other components, a characteristic that has been likened to the impact of wind or motion on the pieces of a mobile.

The analogy of a mobile is useful for considering a second concept in family systems assessment. When piece A of the mobile strikes piece B, piece B may rebound and strike piece A with increased energy. Piece A affects piece B and piece B affects piece A. Circular causality assumes that behavior is reciprocal; each family member's behavior influences the others. If mother responds angrily to her toddler because he turned on the hot water tap while her infant was in the tub, the toddler reciprocates with a response that further influences the mother. It is important to remain open to the multiple interpretations of reality within a family, recognizing that family members may not fully realize how their behavior affects others or how others affect them.

All systems have boundaries. Knowledge of the family's boundaries may enable the nurse to predict the level of social support that the family may perceive and receive. Families with rigid, closed boundaries may have few contacts with the community suprasystem and may require tremendous assistance to network appropriately for help. Conversely, families with very loose, permeable boundaries may be caught between many opinions as they seek to make health-related decisions. Members within family systems may similarly experience extremely closed or permeable boundaries. In enmeshed families, boundaries between parent and child subsystems may be blurred to the extent that children adopt inappropriate parental roles. In more rigid families, the boundaries between adult and child subsystems may be so closed that the developing child is unable to assume more mature roles.

Families attempt to maintain balances between change and stability. The crisis of illness may temporarily produce a state of great change within a family. Efforts at stability, such as emphatic attempts at maintenance of usual feeding routines during the illness of an infant, may seem paradoxical to the period of change; however, both change and stability can and do coexist in family systems. Overwhelming change or rigid equilibrium can contribute to and be symptomatic of severe family dysfunction. Sustained change usually produces a new level of balance as the family regroups and reorganizes to cope with the change.

Stages in Family Development

Change and stability are integral concepts in development. Like individuals, families experience a developmental sequence, which can be divided into eight distinct stages.

Stage One: Marriage (Joining of Families)

Marriage involves the combining of families of origin as well as of individuals. The establishment of couple identity and the negotiation of new relationships with the families of origin is essential to the successful resolution of this stage. The new relationships will vary with the cultural context of the couple.

Stage Two: Families with Infants

This stage begins with the birth of the first child and involves integration of the infant into the family, design and acceptance of new roles, and maintenance of the spousal relationship. The birth of an infant brings about profound changes to the family and offers more challenges than any other stage in family development. A decrease in marital satisfaction is common during this stage, especially if the infant is ill or has a handicapping condition, and is influenced by individual characteristics of the parents, relationships within the nuclear and extended families, and division of labor.

Stage Three: Families with Preschoolers

Stage three begins when the eldest child is 3 years of age and involves socialization of the child(ren) and successful adjustment to separation by parents and child(ren).

Stage Four: Families with School-Aged Children

This stage begins when the eldest child begins elementary or primary school (at about 6 years). Although all stages are perceived by some families as especially stressful, others report this as a particularly stressful stage. Tasks involve establishment of peer relationships by the children and adjustment to peer and other external influences by the parents.

Stage Five: Families with Teenagers

This stage begins when the eldest child is 13 years of age and is viewed by some as an intense period of turmoil. Stage five focuses on the increasing autonomy and individuation of the child, a return to midlife and career issues for parents, and increasing recognition by parents of their predicament as the "sandwich generation."

Stage Six: Families as Launching Centers

Stage six begins when the first child leaves home and continues until the youngest child departs. During this time, the couple realigns the marital relationship while they and the child(ren) adjust to new roles as parents and separate adults.

Stage Seven: Middle-Aged Families

Stage seven begins when the last child leaves home and continues until a parent retires. (This is often a stage for maximum contact between the marriage partners.) Successful resolution depends on development of independent interests within a newly reconstituted couple identity, inclusion of new and extended family relationships, and coming to terms with disabilities and deaths in the older generation. Within some cultures, such as the Vietnamese culture, parents may be incorporated into a multigenerational household.

Stage Eight: Aging Families

This stage begins with retirement and ends with the death of the spouses. It is marked by concern with development of retirement roles, maintenance of individual/couple relationships with aging, and preparation for death.

Tasks and Characteristics of Stepfamilies

Stepfamilies face unique challenges as they attempt to build a new family unit from members who all bring a history of relationships, expectations, and life experiences. Intense conflict may arise as marriage partners attempt to cope with instant children without the benefit of instant affection. The parents move from a fantasy stage, where they dream of fixing everything that went wrong in previous marriages, to a reality stage where the challenges and losses of transition are realized.

Guidelines for Communicating with Families

■ Display a sincere sense of warmth, caring, and encouragement.
■ Demonstrate neutrality; perceptions of partiality toward par-

ticular family members may interfere with assessment and assistance.

- Use active and reflective listening.
- Convey a sense of cooperation and partnership with the family.
- Promote participatory decision making.
- Promote the competencies of the family.
- Encourage the family's use of natural support networks.

Assessment of the Family

Assessment of the family usually involves the entire family, except when the infant or child is too ill to participate.

Assessment	Findings
Internal Structure	
Use a genogram (see Chapter 2) to diagram family structure. The genogram is often useful in helping the family to clarify information related to family composition.	
Family composition	
Refers to everyone in the household.	Extended families and multigenerational households are common among many cultures such as Vietnamese, Chinese, and South Asians.
Ask who is in the family.	**Clinical Alert**
	Losses or additions to families may result in crisis.
Rank order	
Refers to the arrangement of children according to age and gender.	Family position is thought to influence relationships and even careers. Eldest children are considered more conscientious, perfectionistic; middle children are sometimes considered nonconformist, and to have many friends; and youngest children are sometimes seen as precocious, less responsible with resources, and playful.

Assessment	Findings
	Clinical Alert
	Frequent references to rank order ("She's the eldest") may signify a role assignment that is uncomfortable for the individual who is involved.
	The first child can be at increased risk for abuse in abusive families.
Subsystems	**Clinical Alert**
Smaller units in the family marked by sex, role, interests, or age.	A child who acts as a parent surrogate may signify family dysfunction or abuse.
Ask if the family has special smaller groups.	Mothers who are highly involved with their infants and who form tight subsystems with the infants can unintentionally push the father to an outside position. This can exacerbate marital dissatisfaction and conflict.
Boundaries	Strength of boundaries may be influenced by culture. East Indian families, for example, tend to be close-knit and highly interdependent. Cambodians and Laotians consider family problems very personal, private, and off limits to outsiders.
Refers to who is part of what system or subsystem.	
Need to consider if family boundaries and subsystems are closed, open, rigid, or permeable.	
	Clinical Alert
Ask who the family members approach with concerns.	A family with rigid boundaries may become distanced or disengaged from others. Disengagement may also occur within families; these families are characterized by little intrafamilial communication and highly autonomous members.

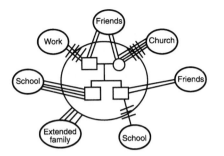
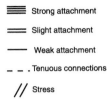

Figure 3-1
Ecomap.

Assessment	Findings
External Structure	
Can be visually represented with an ecomap (Figure 3-1).	Absent or poor social networks, or isolation may indicate family dysfunction.
Culture Way of life for a group. Ask if other languages are spoken. Ask how long family has lived in area/country. Ask if family identifies with a particular ethnic group. Ask how ethnic background influences their lifestyle. Ask what they believe causes health/illness. Ask what they do to prevent/ treat illness. May impact significantly on care.	The internal and external structures of a family, as well as parenting practices, are affected by ethnicity. For example, Native American Indians discipline through observational learning rather than through coercive control.
Religion Influences family values and beliefs. May affect care of the child/ infant.	In families who are Jehovah's Witnesses, blood transfusions are not allowed. Christian Scientists believe that healing

Assessment	Findings
Ask if family is involved in a church or if they identify with a particular religious group. Ask how religion is a part of their life. Observe for religious icons and artifacts in the home.	is a religious function and oppose drugs, blood transfusions, and extensive physical examinations. Buddhists may be reluctant to consent to treatments on holy days.
Social class status and mobility Mold family values. Inquire about work moves, satisfaction, and aspirations.	**Clinical Alert** Family dysfunction may be associated with job instability.
Environment Refers to home, neighborhood, and community. Refers to adequacy and safety of home, school, recreation, and transportation. May affect family's abilities to visit and ongoing care.	**Clinical Alert** Chipped paint, heavy street traffic, uncertain water supplies, and sanitation can all affect family health.
Extended family Refers to families of origin and steprelatives. Ask about contacts (who? frequency? significance?) with extended family members.	Extended family may need to be involved in care if contact is significant. In some cultures (East Indian, Iranian, Japanese), extended family may be consulted about health care decisions.
Family development Use age and school placement of oldest child to delineate stage. Questions evolve from the developmental stage of the family. For stage two, the practitioner might inquire about the differences noticed since the birth of an infant.	**Clinical Alert** A family that resists change may become stuck in a stage. The adolescent, for example, may be treated as a young child, producing great distress. Family breakdown and divorce affect the family differently depending on the timing in the family cycle.

Assessment	Findings
Instrumental functioning Refers to the routine mechanics of eating, dressing, sleeping. Inquire about concerns with accomplishment of daily tasks. In families with young infants, inquire about how childcare and household tasks are shared. Inquire about what families would like to change related to sharing of tasks and responsibilities, if anything.	**Clinical Alert** An ill or disabled child may significantly alter the family's pattern of activities and abilities to carry out activities. Imbalances in the division of labor in families with young infants may be a significant source of stress and conflict.
Expressive functioning Refers to the affective issues and is useful in delineating functional families and those families who are experiencing distress and who would benefit from intervention or referral.	**Clinical Alert** A family may refuse to show emotion appropriately or allow members to do so, which can suggest dysfunction. In alcoholic families, for example, members may show an unusually bland response to extremes in circumstances or behavior. Expression of emotions may be influenced by culture. In some cultures (e.g., Japanese), expression of emotions may be restrained.
Emotional communication Range and type of emotions expressed in a family. Inquire how intense emotions, such as anger and sadness, are expressed and who is most expressive. Ask who provides comfort in the family. When something new is to be tried, who provides support?	**Clinical Alert** Expression may be narrow, rigid, and inappropriate in dysfunctional families.

Assessment	Findings

Verbal communication

Clinical Alert

Verbal communication addresses the clarity, directness, openness and direction of communication.

Can be observed during the interview. Indirect communication may be clarified by asking questions such as "What is your mom telling you?"

Observe congruence of verbal and nonverbal communications.

Observe if family members wait to speak until others are through.

Do parents or older siblings talk down to younger children?

Alcoholic and/or abusive families are frequently characterized by secrecy among family members and in relation to those outside the family. Within dysfunctional families, verbal exchanges may evidence blaming, scapegoating, or derogatory remarks. Adolescents may be exposed to public ridicule, threats related to expulsion from the family and to forced encounters with police, and intense criticism.

Triangulation refers to an indirect communication pattern in which one member communicates with another through a third member.

Circular communications

Reciprocal communications that are adaptive or maladaptive.

Useful in understanding communications in dyads.

If a mother complains that her adolescent never listens to her, you might inquire: "So Susan ignores your instruction. What do you do then?"

Problem solving

Decision making is culturally influenced. In many cultures (e.g., Hispanic, Vietnamese, Puerto Rican) the father is the main family decision maker.

Assessment	Findings
Refers to ability of family to solve own problems.	**Clinical Alert**
Ask who first notices problems, how decisions are made, who makes decisions.	Dysfunctional families may tend to employ a narrow range of strategies or to consistently apply inappropriate strategies.
Roles	**Clinical Alert**
Focuses on established behavior patterns.	Dysfunctional families may assign narrowly prescriptive roles.
Consider flexibility or rigidity of roles and whether certain idiosyncratic roles are applied to family members. ("She's always been a problem"; "He's a good kid").	
Consider the effect of culture on roles. Ask "In your culture what do women do? What do men do?"	
Consider the influence of the multigenerational family on roles. "In your family, what did your father do? What did your mother do?"	
Control	**Clinical Alert**
Refers to ways of influencing the behavior of others. May be psychological (use of communication and feelings), corporal (hugging or spanking), or instrumental (use of reinforcers such as privileges or objects).	Excessive control or chaos in relation to rules may signify an abusive family.
Inquire about family rules and what occurs when rules are broken.	
Ask who enforces family rules.	

Assessment	Findings
Do children have a say in rules?	
Consider the impact of culture on family expectations. Ask "How are children expected to behave? What happens if they do not behave?"	
Alliances/coalitions	**Clinical Alert**
Refers to balance and intensity of relationships between or among family members.	In sexually abusive families, the father and daughter coalition may supplant the spousal relationship.

Related Nursing Diagnoses

Anxiety: Related to situational crisis; family chaos.

Impaired verbal communication: Related to family processes; family roles; inadequate progression of family life cycle.

Decisional conflict: Related to differing expectations about family roles and responsibilities.

Parental role conflict: Related to ineffective communication, differing expectations, influences of extended family.

Compromised family coping: Related to situational crisis; ineffective expressive functioning; social isolation; stress; fatigue; adjustment to chronic health concerns.

Risk for impaired parenting: Related to situational crisis; marital conflict; knowledge deficit; fatigue; stress.

Dysfunctional family processes: Alcoholism.

Interrupted family processes: Related to situational crisis; change in family structure.

Impaired parenting: Related to skill deficit; stress; inadequate progression of family life cycle; marital conflict; fatigue.

Home Visits and Assessments

4

Making home visits and delivering home-based nursing gives the nurse an excellent opportunity to observe and interact with families in an environment that is familiar to them. Further, by visiting the home, the nurse is able to assess safety, hygiene, support systems, and play stimulation within the environment that is closest to the family.

Making Home Visits

In making home visits, it is essential that the nurse recognize his or her status as a visitor in the home with services that the family can accept or reject. The relationship is a negotiated one, and the nurse must recognize that successful negotiation entails gaining support and acceptance from the family.

To gain and maintain access to the home, the nurse needs to demonstrate flexibility, an understanding of the diversity present in homes, and an awareness of social rules that will affect the relationship between the family and nurse. In establishing initial contact with a family, some guidelines assist in ensuring that the contact is successful:

- Identify affiliation, source of referral, purpose of referral, knowledge of situation, and how families may further contact the nurse, with the first telephone call.
- Demonstrate willingness to negotiate times for the visit.
- Ask for clear directions to the home. If the area is unfamiliar, check with a supervisor for more detailed directions.
- Alert the family about when the visit will occur.
- Establish where to park and how to access the home.

Making the Initial Visit

When making the initial visit, family-centered actions will facilitate development of trust and rapport. The nurse must also be aware of variables that will affect assessment and the safety of the nurse:

- Maintain a respectful distance. Do not enter the family's space prematurely. Enter the home and less public areas within the home when verbally and nonverbally invited to do so.
- Respect customs. Place shoes and coat in areas comfortable to the family. Observe for and avoid special areas that certain family members claim for sitting.
- Suspend values. What works for this family may differ from the nurse's perception of what is acceptable.
- Be prepared to accept hospitality; professional boundaries are less secure in home settings, and the relationship may be less formal.
- Be prepared for the unpredictable. Homes can be more distracting than clinical settings; they have no common baseline, and variables are less controlled. Distractions and variations provide useful information for ongoing care and the relationship.
- Priorities need to remain fluid to accommodate differences between the family's perceptions and that of the nurse. Preset nurse agendas are often only a starting point.
- Attend to personal safety. Keep car doors locked and park in a well-lighted area; check surroundings before getting out of the car, do not get out of the car if suspicious behavior is occurring, and assess the safety of the interior environment of the home before entering.
- Establish dates and times for the next visit before leaving.

Assessment of the Home Environment
Safety

Observe for condition of stairs, stairwells, doors, and windows; presence and condition of smoke and CO_2 detectors; source of heat and light; presence of infant gates and locks on cupboards; accessibility of poisonous substances and medications; presence of hanging cords; accessibility of cooking pot handles; nonskid rugs; temperature of water; infant walkers; condition of crib and high chair; presence of needles and drug paraphenalia; presence and storage of firearms; proximity to pools; age and condition of the dwelling. Observe for proximity of dwelling to smelters, battery recycling plants, or other industries likely to release lead.

Hygiene

Observe for cleanliness, storage and handling of perishable foodstuffs (especially meat); handling of pacifiers and bottles; handwashing practices; odors; condition of water supply; type and adequacy of waste disposal; pests; type and condition of clothing worn by family members; and hygiene of family members.

Availability of Transportation and Facilities

Observe for presence of vehicles; bus stops; condition of roads; driveways; distance to nearest neighbor; presence of telephone; and proximity to schools, shopping, recreation, and health care services.

Nutritional Practices

Observe what snack foods are available; cooking odors; accessibility of food for children; availability of choice in menu; and ethnic or religious food observances.

Support Networks

Observe for family pictures and pictures of friends; presence of a telephone and type of calls received; and proximity to neighbors and other family members.

Family Interactions

Observe for spontaneous vocalization between parents and children; verbal responses of parents to vocalizations of children; use of praise with children; demonstrations of affection; use of scolding or shouting; attempts to explain or teach about objects or situations; attempts to look at children, teaching of culturally appropriate rules of behavior, display of children's art/crafts; introduction of children to nurse; and encouragement of age-appropriate independence.

Provision of Stimulation and Opportunities for Rest

Observe for presence of age-appropriate toys and toys with variety; recreational and exercise aids; and books, pets, and television. Observe for amount of time that children spend watching television and interaction of parents in relation to television; areas and space available in the home for privacy; amount of space or crowding evident in home; and adequacy of sleeping facilities.

Religious and Cultural Influences

Observe for presence of religious icons, bibles, art, and cultural artifacts; ethnic cooking utensils; and type of clothing worn by family members.

Related Nursing Diagnoses

Impaired comfort: Related to inadequate heating; inadequate ventilation; inadequate transportation; poor socioeconomic conditions.

Compromised family coping: Related to lack of knowledge of resources; isolation.

Knowledge deficit: Related to hygienic needs; food handling; safety; child care; developmental needs of children; parenting.

Risk for impaired parenting: Related to inappropriate caretaking behaviors; lack of viable social support; lack of knowledge.

Hopelessness: Related to lack of social support; socioeconomic conditions.

Impaired home maintenance: Related to inadequate finances; knowledge deficit, and lack of resources.

Physical Assessment

5

The physical assessment skills are inspection, palpation, percussion, and auscultation. (The sequence in abdominal assessment is inspection, auscultation, percussion, and palpation.) The acquisition of these skills requires patience, practice, and continual refinement. More detail on these skills may be found in a textbook of adult assessment skills.

Guidelines for Inspection

- Inspection is a simple but highly skilled technique.
- Inspection involves the use of sight, hearing, and smell in a systematic assessment of infants and children.
- Inspection is essential at the beginning of the health assessment to detect obvious health concerns and to establish priorities.
- Inspection should be thorough and should involve each area of the body.
- Body parts are assessed for shape, color, symmetry, odor (Table 5-1), and abnormalities.
- Careful inspection requires good lighting.

Guidelines for Palpation

- Palpation involves the use of fingers and palms to determine temperature, hydration, texture, shape, movement, and areas of tenderness.
- Warm hands before beginning palpation.
- Keep fingernails short.
- Palpate areas of tenderness or vulnerability last.
- Palpate with fingertips for pulsation, size, shape, texture, and hydration.
- Palpate with palms for vibration.
- Palpate with back of hand for temperature.

Table 5-1   Significance of Common Body Odors

Odor	Significance
Acetone or fruity odor	May indicate diabetic acidosis
Ammonia	May indicate urinary tract infection
Fecal odor (breath or diaper area)	Associated with soiled diapers, fecal incontinence, bowel obstruction
Foul-smelling stool	May be indicative of gastroenteritis, cystic fibrosis, malabsorption syndromes
Halitosis	Associated with poor oral hygiene, dental caries or abscess, throat infection, sinusitis, constipation, foreign body in nasal passage
Musty odor	Associated with infection underneath a cast or dressing
Sweet, thick odor	May be indicative of *Pseudomonas* infection

- Use conversation or games to relax child during palpation. Muscle guarding related to tension can obscure findings. Observe reactions to palpation rather than asking "Does it hurt?"
- The nurse can assist the ticklish child by first placing the child's hands on the skin and gradually sliding hands over those of the child or by having the child keep his or her hands over the nurse's during examination.
- Move firmly and without hesitation.

Guidelines for Percussion

- Percussion involves the use of tapping to produce sound waves, which are characterized regarding intensity, pitch, duration, and quality (Table 5-2).
- Percussion may be *direct* or *indirect.*
    Direct percussion involves striking the body part directly with one or two fingers.
    Indirect percussion involves a pleximeter and a plexor.
        Place the middle finger (pleximeter) of the *nondominant hand* gently against child's skin.

Table 5-2 Percussion Sounds

Percussion Sound	Intensity	Pitch	Duration	Quality	Body Region Where Sound May Be Heard
Tympany	Loud	High	Moderate	Drumlike	Gastric bubble; air-filled intestine (simulate by tapping puffed out cheeks)
Resonance	Moderate to loud	Low	Long	Hollow	Lungs
Hyperresonance	Very loud	Very low	Long	Booming	Lungs with trapped air; lungs of a young child
Dullness	Soft to moderate	High	Moderate	Thudlike	Liver; fluid-filled space, such as stomach
Flatness	Soft	High	Short	Flat	Muscle

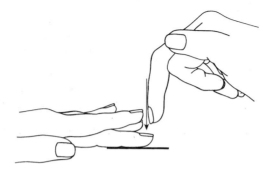

Figure 5-1
Percussion. Note position of fingers.

> Strike the distal joint of the pleximeter with the tip of the
> middle finger (plexor) of the *dominant* hand (Figure 5-1).
> The blow to the pleximeter should be crisp, and the plexor
> must be perpendicular.
> The wrist movement is essential to percussion and must be
> a snapping motion.
> The nail of the plexor should be short.

■ Percuss from resonance to dullness.

Guidelines for Auscultation

■ Auscultation is the process of listening for body sounds.
■ The bell (cupped portion) of the stethoscope is used for
low-pitched sounds (for example, cardiovascular sounds), and
the diaphragm (flat portion) for higher-pitched sounds (for
example, those found in the lung and bowel).
■ The stethoscope is placed firmly against the wall of the body
part. The examiner must avoid pressing too firmly, causing the
skin to flatten and vibrations to decrease. Resting the heel of the
hand on the child will assist in avoiding heavy pressure.
■ The examiner should practice in identifying normal sounds
before trying to identify abnormal ones.

Preparation for Examination

6

Preparation of Environment

- Try to perform assessments somewhere other than in the child's "safe areas," when possible. "Safe areas" include the child's bedside or play area.
- Place toys, bright posters, and motifs in the examination room or area to make it look less threatening to the child.
- Limit number of people in room and number of people entering and leaving the area.
- Set air conditioner on low because noisy fans can interfere with auscultation.
- Eliminate drafts from the examining area. Cold is uncomfortable for the infant or child who is minimally dressed and can alter findings. A child who is cold may appear mottled, which can also signify cardiac or respiratory disease.
- Provide privacy for school-aged children and adolescents.

Preparation of Equipment

- Ensure that all equipment is readily available.
- Place threatening or strange equipment out of easy view before beginning examination of the young child.
- Warm hands and equipment before starting examination. Equipment can be warmed with hands or with warm water.

Equipment for Physical Assessment

Cotton-tipped applicators
Paper towels and tissue
Disposable pads
Drapes

Gown for child
Gloves
Lubricant
Scale for weight
Measuring board or measuring tray
Tape measure
Stethoscope
Pediatric blood pressure cuff
Sphygmomanometer
Thermometers (rectal and oral)
Tongue depressor
Flashlight
Otoscope
Ophthalmoscope
Eye chart
Percussion hammer
Safety pins
Wristwatch with second hand
Physical assessment forms
Denver II Screening Test

Guidelines for Physical Assessment of Infant or Child

■ Perform a general head-to-toe assessment while collecting the health history and the vital signs. General assessment assists in establishing priorities. Note obvious areas of distress. For example, if a child is experiencing pronounced respiratory problems, assessment of this area is a priority.

■ Physical assessment is an essential component of nursing care. Children often cannot tell the caregiver what is wrong. The caregiver must be able to assess and to communicate concerns of the child arising from the assessment.

■ Some aspects of a complete physical examination may be omitted during the daily assessment, depending on the child's age, health status, and the reason for the health care contact. Examples of assessments that need not always be included are height, head circumference, weight, deep tendon reflexes, and neurologic tests.

■ An orderly, systematic, head-to-toe approach to examination may not be possible; it is often necessary to vary the sequence to fit the child. *Flexibility is essential;* however, all necessary aspects of an examination must eventually be covered.

■ Often several observations can be made at once because of the size of the area being examined. For example, while checking respiratory rate it is possible to observe the type and quality of respirations, the presence or absence of retractions, the color of the trunk, and whether there is a heave under the nipple.

■ Perform as much of the examination as possible with the child in a sitting position because lying down may cause the child to feel more vulnerable.

■ Perform the least distressing aspects of the examination first. What is distressing for one age-group may not be for another age-group.

■ Where possible, use gaming, puppets, and dolls to ease the anxiety of younger children.

■ Use a kind, firm, direct approach. Tell the child what to do rather than asking for cooperation. Demonstration assists with compliance.

■ Examine painful areas last in sequence.

■ Allow children to handle the equipment and provide time for play, anticipatory guidance before beginning the examination.

■ Use both hands when possible. One hand or probing fingers may be construed as intrusive.

■ Do not leave infants and children unattended on an examining room table.

Age-Related Approaches to Physical Assessment
Infant (1 to 12 Months)

■ Approach the infant quietly, gently. Excessive smiling, loud voices, and rapid movements may frighten infants.

■ Remove all clothes, except for the diaper of a male child.

■ Allow the infant to be held by the parent for as much of the examination as possible.

■ Distract the infant with bright toys, peek-a-boo games, and talking.

■ Vary the sequence of the assessment with the infant's activity level. If the infant is quiet, obtain the pulse and respiratory rates and auscultate the lungs, heart, and abdomen at the beginning of the examination.

- Obtain the temperature and perform other intrusive examinations (throat, ear, blood pressure) at the end of the examination.
- The parent can assist, if willing, with assessment of the ears and mouth.

Toddler (12 Months to 3 Years)

- Approach the toddler gradually. Keep physical contact to a minimum until the toddler is acquainted with you.
- Allow the toddler to remain near the parent or to be held by the parent, whenever possible.
- Introduce and use equipment gradually.
- Allow the child to handle the equipment.
- Use play to approach the child. If the child remains upset and apprehensive, carry out the assessment as quickly as possible.
- Expose the child minimally. Appropriate clothing should be removed immediately before specific assessments, and preferably by the parent.
- Sequencing of the assessment is similar to that recommended for the infant.
- Encourage use of comfort objects such as blankets and stuffed toys.
- Tell the child when the assessment is completed.
- Praise the child for cooperation.

Preschool-Aged Child (3 to 6 Years)

- Allow the child to remain close to the parent.
- Allow the child to handle the equipment. Demonstrations of equipment are useful: "You can hear your own heartbeat."
- Expose the child minimally. Allow the child to take off own clothes. *This age-group is particularly modest.*
- Use games to gain cooperation: "Let's see how far you can stick out your tongue."
- Tell a story or perform a simple trick to relieve apprehension.

School-Aged Child (6 to 12 Years)

- Give the older child the choice about whether the parent is present during assessment.
- Allow the child to remove own clothing.
- Give the child a gown.
- Explain purposes of equipment: "The stethoscope is used to listen to your heartbeat."

Adolescent (12 Years and Older)

- Give the adolescent the choice about whether the parent is present.
- Allow the adolescent to undress in private.
- Give time for the adolescent to regain self-composure before beginning the examination.
- Explain the purposes of the equipment and of assessments.
- Emphasize normalcy of development.
- Give feedback about assessment findings during examination, if appropriate. If in doubt about whether the sharing of particular information is appropriate, check with a more experienced caregiver.
- Make comments about sexual development in a matter-of-fact fashion.

Dimensions of Nutritional Assessment

7

Rationale

Nutritional assessment is an important initial step in nursing care and in preventive health care. It aids in identifying eating practices, misconceptions, and symptoms that can lead to nutritional problems. Because the nurse often has continued contact with the parents and child, the nurse can often influence dietary practices.

Establishing Weight

Weight measurement is plotted on a growth chart (see Appendix B). Normally weight remains within the same percentile from measurement to measurement. Sudden increases or decreases should be noted. Average weight and height increases for each age are summarized in Table 7-1.

Measurement of Weight	Significance of Findings
Infants (1 to 12 months)	
Undress completely (including diaper) and lay on a balance infant scale. Protect the scale surface with a cloth or paper liner. Place hand lightly above the infant for safety. If precise measurements are required, have a second nurse perform an independent	Breast-fed infants tend to display slower growth than bottle-fed infants, especially in the second half of the first year. **Clinical Alert** Weight loss or failure to gain weight may be related to dehydration, acute infections,

Table 7-1 Physical Growth During Infancy and Childhood

Age	Weight	Height
0 to 6 months	Average weekly gain 140-200 gm (5-7 oz) Birth weight doubles by 4-6 mo	Average monthly gain 2.5 cm (1 in)
6 to 18 months	Average weekly gain 85-140 gm (3-5 oz) Birth weight triples by 1 year	Average monthly gain 1.25 cm (0.5 in)
18 months to 3 years	Average yearly gain 2-3 kg (4.4-6.6 lb)	Height at 2 years approximately half of adult height
1-2 years		Average gain 12 cm (4.8 in)
2-3 years		Average gain 6-8 cm (2.4-3.2 in)
3 to 6 years	Average yearly gain 1.8-2.7 kg (4-6 lb)	Yearly gain 6-8 cm (2.4-3.2 in)
6 to 12 years	Average yearly gain 1.8-2.7 kg (4-6 lb)	Yearly gain 5 cm (2 in)
Girl, 10 to 14 years	Average gain 17.5 kg (38.5 lb)	95% of adult height achieved by onset of menarche Average gain 20.5 cm (8.1 in)
Boy, 12 to 16 years	Average gain 23.7 kg (52.1 lb)	95% of adult height achieved by 15 years Average gain 27.5 cm (11 in)

Measurement of Weight	Significance of Findings

measurement. If there is a difference between the two measurements, a third one should be performed. When possible, use the same scale for subsequent weight measurements.

Toddlers and Preschoolers (12 months to 6 years)

Undress, except for underpants, and weigh on a standing, balance scale. (Children younger than 2 years are weighed on an infant or sitting scale unless they can stand well.)

Older Children (6 Years and Older)

Remove shoes. Weigh clothed, on a standing scale.

feeding disorders, malabsorption, chronic disease, neglect, excessive ingestion of apple and pear juices, thyroid disorders, ectodermal dysplasias, diabetes, anorexia nervosa, cocaine use by mother in prenatal period, fetal alcohol syndrome, tuberculosis, or acquired immune deficiency syndrome (AIDS). A loss of 10% on a growth chart is indicative of severe weight loss. Excessive weight gain may be related to chronic renal, pulmonary, or cardiovascular disorders or to endocrine dysfunction. Children who are 120% or more of ideal body weight for height and age are considered obese.

Clinical Alert

Marked weight loss is often an initial sign of Type 1 diabetes. A body weight of less than 85% of the expected norm in adolescents may signal anorexia nervosa, especially if bradycardia, cold intolerance, dry skin, brittle nails, body distortion, and preoccupation with food are present. Weight loss may also accompany amphetamine use.

Establishing Height

Measurement of Height/Length	Significance of Findings

Infants/Toddlers
(1 to 24 months)

Lay infant flat. Have parent hold infant's head as the infant's legs are extended and pushed *gently* toward the table. Measure the distance between marks made indicating heel tips (with toes pointing toward the ceiling) and vertex of head. *Do not use a cloth tape* for measurement because it may stretch. If using a measuring board or tray, align the infant's head against the top bar and ask the parent to secure the infant's head there. Straighten the infant's body and, while holding the feet in a vertical position, bring the foot board snugly up against the bottom of the feet.

Use the same technique to obtain subsequent height measurements.

Clinical Alert

Although short stature is usually genetically predetermined, it may also indicate chronic heart or renal disease, growth hormone deficiency, malnutrition, Kearns-Sayre syndrome, Turner's syndrome and dwarfism, methadone exposure, or fetal alcohol syndrome.

Children (24 Months and Older)

Have child, in stocking feet or bare feet, stand straight on a standard scale, and measure with the attached marker, to the nearest 0.1 cm (0.03 in).

Height is usually less in the afternoon than in the morning. Correct for this tendency by placing slight upward pressure under the jaw.

Measurement of Height/Length	Significance of Findings

If a scale with a measuring bar is not available or if a child is afraid of standing on the scale's base, have the child stand erect against a wall. Place a flat object, such as a clipboard, on the child's head, at right angles to the wall. Read the height at the point where the flat object touches the measuring tape or the wall-mounted unit (stadiometer).

Assessment of Eating Practices

Assessment of eating practices requires sensitivity on the part of the nurse. Eating practices are highly personal, and cultural, and can be more accurately assessed once a rapport has been established. Guilt, apprehension, and a desire to give the "right" responses can alter the accuracy of the assessment.

Table 7-2 lists eating habits typical of various age-groups.

General Assessment

■ Is your child on a special diet?
■ Are there any suspected or known food allergies?
■ Describe your child's typical intake over 24 hours (what child ate for each meal and between meals).
■ Has your child lost or gained weight recently?
■ Do any cultural, ethnic, or religious influences affect your child's diet? How?
■ Do you have any concerns?

Assessment of Feeding Practices of Infants

■ How much weight did you (mother) gain during pregnancy?
■ What was your infant's birth weight? When did it double? triple?
■ What vitamin supplements does your infant receive?

Table 7-2 Eating Habits and Concerns Common to Various Age-Groups

Age-Group	Eating Practices	Concerns Arising from Eating Practices
Infants/Toddlers (1 to 18 months)	Formula or breast milk forms major part of diet for first 6 months and is generally recommended until 1 year. Solid foods assume greater importance in second 6 months of life. By 1 year, infant is able to eat all solid foods unless food intolerance develops. White grape juice is a healthy form of juice. Juice intake should be limited to no more than 150 ml per day in infants.	Mothers may feed child in accordance with practices followed in their own upbringing. Early introduction of solid foods (before 5 or 6 months) may contribute to allergies. Sensitivity to cow's milk may be suggested by colic, sleeplessness, diarrhea, abdominal pain, chronic nasal discharge, recurrent respiratory ailments, eczema, pallor, and excessive crying. Colic, regurgitation, diarrhea, constipation, bottle mouth syndrome, and rashes are common concerns associated with infant feeding. Yellowish skin coloration may accompany persistent feeding of carrots. Excess milk intake in later infancy may lead to milk anemia. Excessive ingestion of pear and apple juices may be associated with failure to thrive, tooth decay, diarrhea, and obesity.

Continued

Table 7-2   Eating Habits and Concerns Common to Various Age-Groups—cont'd

Age-Group	Eating Practices	Concerns Arising from Eating Practices
Toddlers/Preschool-Aged Children (18 months to 6 years)	Appetites tend to be erratic because of sporadic energy needs. Appetites of toddlers and preschoolers are smaller than those of infants because of slowed growth. Toddlers and preschoolers have definite likes and dislikes. Likes include foods such as yogurt, fruit drinks, fruit breads, and cookies that are easy to eat and to handle. Dislikes include casseroles, liver, and cooked vegetables. Food is often consumed "on the go." Children may go on "food jags," where one food is preferred for a few days. Variety is desirable, but not necessary so long as the child eats from all food groups during the course of a day.	Some children may snack their way through the day and rarely consume a regular meal. Mealtimes may become a battle between parents and toddlers over types and amounts of food eaten. Parents may express concern over toddlers' or preschoolers' diminished appetite. Eighty percent of children with both parents obese are likely to be obese. It is recommended that children by 2 years of age receive baseline screening for cardiovascular disease factors such as parental obesity, age and weight, and blood pressure measures.

School-Aged Children (6 to 12 years)	Children generally have a good appetite and like variety.	Parents may express concern over table manners.
	Plain foods still preferred.	
	Increasing numbers of activities compete with mealtimes.	
	Television and peers influence food choices.	
Adolescents (12 years and older)	Food habits include skipping meals (especially breakfast), carbonated drinks, fast foods, snacking, and unusual food choices.	Alcohol may form substantial portion of caloric intake.
	Adolescents consume increasingly larger amounts of alcohol at younger ages.	Preoccupation with food and feelings of guilt may be indicative of eating disorders. Anorexia nervosa and bulimia are serious disorders related to obsession to lose weight.
	Adolescent girls frequently are calorie conscious and may diet, thus severely restricting their calcium intake.	Low calcium intake may place adolescent females at risk for osteoporosis.

- Do you give your infant extra fluids such as juice or water?
- At what age did you start cereals, vegetables, fruits, meat (or other sources of proteins), table foods, and finger foods?
- Does your infant spit up frequently? What are her/his stools like?
- Does your infant have any problems with feeding (for example, lethargy, poor sucking, regurgitation, colic, irritability, rash, diarrhea)?
- Breast-fed infants
    How long does your infant feed at one time?
    Do you alternate breasts?
    How do you recognize that your infant is hungry? Full?
    Describe your infant's elimination and sleeping patterns.
    Describe your usual daily diet.
    Do you have concerns related to breast-feeding?
- Formula-fed infants
    What type of formula is your infant on?
    How do you prepare the formula?
    What type of bottle does your infant take?
    How many ounces (ml) of formula does your infant drink in a day?
    Do you prop or hold your infant while feeding?
    Do you have concerns related to bottle-feeding?

Assessment of Feeding Practices of Toddlers and Children

- What foods does your child prefer? Dislike?
- Does the child snack? If so, when? What foods are given as snacks? When are sweet foods eaten?
- What assistance does your child require with eating?

Assessment of Feeding Practices of Adolescents

- What foods do you prefer? Dislike?
- What foods do you choose for a snack?
- Are you satisfied with the quantity and kinds of food you eat?
- Have you tried to change your food intake? In what ways?
- Do you fast or use other weight control measures?
- Have you started your menstrual periods (girls)? Are you taking an oral contraceptive?

- How active are you in sports or fitness activities?
- What exercise regimens do you follow?

Assessment of Physical Signs of Nutrition or Malnutrition

Many of the assessments related to nutritional status can be combined with other areas of the physical assessment. Table 7-3 outlines the head-to-toe observations that provide information about a child's nutritional status.

Related Nursing Diagnoses

Risk for activity intolerance: Related to fatigue; inadequate protein and calories; electrolyte imbalance.

Risk for constipation: Related to formula intake; excess intake of calcium; decreased intake of fiber.

Diarrhea: Related to deficiency of niacin; excess vitamin C; food intolerances; excess consumption of fresh fruit or other high-fiber foods; excess consumption of juices.

Decreased cardiac output: Related to excess intake of niacin, potassium; inadequate intake of magnesium, potassium.

Impaired dentition: Related to decreased intake of calcium; increased intake of carbonated drinks; increased intake of fruit juices; vitamin A, C, or D deficiencies; fluoride excess; improper bottle-feeding practices.

Deficient fluid volume: Related to inadequate intake of fluids; excessive loss of fluids secondary to diarrhea or vomiting (physiologic or self-induced).

Delayed growth and development: Related to deficit of protein and calories; genetic endowment; malabsorption.

Ineffective health maintenance: Related to lack of knowledge; alcohol abuse; skin lesions; dental caries; obesity; anorexia; bowel irregularity; inappropriate weight control measures (self-induced vomiting, diuretic and laxative abuse).

Deficient knowledge: Related to management of an age-appropriate diet; effects of overly restrictive dietary regimens.

Nutrition: Less than body requirements related to lack of knowledge of adequate nutrition; crash or fad diets; anorexia; nausea and vomiting; allergy; congenital anomalies; growth spurts; inability to procure food.

Text continued on p. 71

Table 7-3 Physical Assessment of Nutrition

Body Area	Signs of Adequate/Appropriate Nutrition	Signs of Inadequate/Inappropriate Nutrition	Possible Causes of Inadequate/Inappropriate Nutrition
General growth	Height, weight, head circumference within 5th and 95th percentiles	Height, weight, head circumference below or above 5th and 95th percentiles	Protein, fats, vitamin A, niacin, calcium, iodine, manganese, zinc deficiency/excess
	Sexual development age appropriate	Delayed sexual maturation	Less than expected growth possibly related to disease (especially endocrine dysfunction) or to genetic endowment
			Vitamin A or D excess
Skin	Elastic, firm, slightly dry; no lesions, rashes, hyperpigmentation	Dryness	Vitamin A deficiency
			Essential and unsaturated fatty acid deficiency
		Swollen red pigmentation (pellagrous dermatosis)	Niacin deficiency
		Hyperpigmentation	Vitamin B_{12}, folic acid, niacin deficiency
		Edema	Protein deficiency or sodium excess
		Poor skin turgor	Water, sodium deficiency
		Petechiae	Ascorbic acid deficiency
		Delayed wound healing	Vitamin C deficiency
		Decreased subcutaneous tissue	Prolonged caloric deficiency
		Pallor	Iron, vitamin B_{12} or C, folic acid, pyridoxine deficiency

Hair	Shiny, firm, elastic	Dull, dry, thin, brittle, sparse, easily plucked	Protein, caloric deficiency
		Alopecia	Protein, caloric, or zinc deficiency
Head	Head evenly molded, with occipital prominence; facial features symmetric	Skull flattened, frontal bones prominent	Vitamin D deficiency
	Sutures fused by 12 to 18 months	Suture fusion delayed	Vitamin D deficiency
		Hard, tender lumps in occipital region	Vitamin A excess
		Headache	Thiamine excess
Neck	Thyroid gland not obvious to inspection, palpable in midline	Thyroid gland enlarged, obvious to inspection	Iodine deficiency
Eyes	Clear, bright, shiny	Dull, soft cornea; white or gray spots on cornea (Bitot's spots)	Vitamin A deficiency
	Membranes pink and moist	Pale membranes	Iron deficiency
		Burning, itching, photophobia	Riboflavin deficiency
	Night vision adequate	Nightblindness	Vitamin A deficiency
		Redness, fissuring at corners of eyes	Riboflavin, niacin deficiency

Continued

Table 7-3   Physical Assessment of Nutrition—cont'd

Body Area	Signs of Adequate/ Appropriate Nutrition	Signs of Inadequate/ Inappropriate Nutrition	Possible Causes of Inadequate/ Inappropriate Nutrition
Nose	Smooth, intact nasal angle	Cracks, irritation at nasal angle	Niacin deficiency, vitamin A excess
Lips	Smooth, moist, no edema	Angular fissures, redness and edema	Riboflavin deficiency, vitamin A excess
Tongue	Deep pink, papillae visible, moist, taste sensation, no edema	Paleness	Iron deficiency
		Red, swollen, raw	Folic acid, niacin, vitamin B or B_{12} deficiency
		Magenta coloration	Riboflavin deficiency
		Diminished taste	Zinc deficiency
Gums	Firm, coral color	Spongy, bleed easily, receding	Ascorbic acid deficiency
Teeth	White, smooth, free of spots or pits	Mottled enamel, brown spots, pits	Fluoride excess, or discoloration from antibiotics
		Defective enamel	Vitamin A, C, or D, or calcium, phosphorus deficiency
		Caries	Carbohydrate excess, poor hygiene

Cardiovascular system	Pulse and blood pressure within normal limits for age	Palpitations	Thiamine deficiency
		Rapid pulse	Potassium deficiency
		Arrhythmia	Niacin, potassium excess; magnesium, potassium deficiency
		High blood pressure	Sodium excess
		Decreased blood pressure	Thiamine deficiency
		Constipation	Calcium excess, overrigid toilet training, inadequate intake of high-fiber foods or fluids
Gastrointestinal system	Bowel habits normal for age	Diarrhea	Niacin deficiency; vitamin C excess; high consumption of fresh fruit, other high-fiber foods, excessive consumption of juices

Continued

Table 7-3 Physical Assessment of Nutrition—cont'd

Body Area	Signs of Adequate/ Appropriate Nutrition	Signs of Inadequate/ Inappropriate Nutrition	Possible Causes of Inadequate/ Inappropriate Nutrition
Musculoskeletal system	Muscles firm and well developed, joints flexible and pain free, extremities symmetric and straight, spinal nerves normal	Muscles atrophied, dependent edema	Protein, caloric deficiency
		Knock-knee, bowleg, epiphyseal enlargement	Vitamin D deficiency; disease processes
		Bleeding into joints, pain	Vitamin C deficiency
		Beading on ribs	Vitamins C and D deficiency
Neurologic system	Behavior alert and responsive, intact muscle innervation	Listlessness, irritability, lethargy	Thiamine, niacin, pyridoxine, iron, protein, caloric deficiency
		Tetany	Magnesium deficiency
		Convulsions	Thiamine, pyridoxine, vitamin D, calcium deficiency, phosphorus excess
		Unsteadiness, numbness in hands and feet	Pyridoxine excess
		Diminished reflexes	Thiamine deficiency

Nutrition: More than body requirements related to lack of basic nutritional knowledge; ethnic or family values.

Disturbed body image: Related to obesity.

Sexual dysfunction: Secondary to obesity; alcohol abuse.

Effective breast-feeding: Related to knowledge; support.

Ineffective breast-feeding: Related to knowledge; lack of support.

MEASUREMENT OF VITAL SIGNS

II

Body Temperature, Pulse, and Respirations

8

Nursing fundamentals textbooks provide comprehensive discussions of measurement of vital signs. Only significant pediatric variations in the measurement of temperature, pulse, and respirations are presented here.

Measurement of Body Temperature
Rationale

Environmental factors and relatively minor infections can produce a much higher temperature in infants and young children than would be expected in older children and adults. In most cases, an elevated temperature is the result of fever and is one of the most common manifestations of illness in young children. In very young infants, fever may be one of the few signs of an underlying disorder. In toddlers, febrile convulsions can parallel fever and are of particular concern. The absence or presence of fever and the cause of fever are important in planning nursing care. Body temperature should be measured on admission to the health care facility, before and after surgery or invasive diagnostic procedures, during the course of an unidentified infection, after fever reduction measures have been taken, and any time that an infant or child looks flushed, feels warm, or is lethargic.

Anatomy and Physiology

Temperature is regulated from within the hypothalamus. During an infection, the body's normal set point is elevated, and the

Table 8-1   Body Temperature in Well Children

Age	Temperature	
	°C	°F
3 mo	37.5	99.4
1 yr	37.7	99.7
3 yr	37.2	99.0
5 yr	37.0	98.6
7 yr	36.8	98.3
9 yr	36.7	98.1
13 yr	36.6	97.8

Modified from Lowrey GH: *Growth and development of children,* ed 8, St Louis, 1986, Mosby.

hypothalamus increases heat production until the body's core temperature is consistent with this new set point. Shivering and vasoconstriction during the chill phase help the body reach the new set point by conserving and generating heat.

The temperature-regulating mechanisms in infants and young children are not well developed, and dramatic fluctuations can occur. A young child's temperature may vary as much as 1.6° C (3° F) in a single day. Fluctuations are less apparent as temperature-regulating mechanisms mature.

The control of body heat loss increases with age. The ability of muscles to shiver increases with maturity, and the child will accumulate ever greater amounts of adipose tissue necessary for insulation against heat loss. Heat production decreases with age. The infant produces relatively more heat per unit of body weight than the adult does, as reflected by the infant's higher average body temperature (Table 8-1). A variety of other factors also affect the body temperature of the child (Table 8-2).

Preparation

Ask the parent or child if the child has been febrile, and if so, whether the fever has followed a pattern. Sustained fevers show little fluctuation and are found in children with scarlet fever or central nervous system disorders. Intermittent fevers, with wide variations in body temperature, occur with bacteremia or viremia. Recurrent fevers occur with Hodgkin's disease. Late afternoon

Table 8-2   Factors Influencing Body Temperature

Factor	Effect
Active exercise	May temporarily raise temperature
Stress, crying	Raises body temperature
Diurnal variation	Body temperature is lowest between 0100 and 0400 hours (1:00 and 4:00 AM), highest between 1600 and 1800 hours (4:00 and 6:00 PM)
Environment, including clothing, swaddling, and nesting	Body temperature can vary with room temperature, amount and type of clothing
Pharmacologic agents (muscle relaxants, vasodilating anesthetic agents)	Decrease body temperature

elevations with a return to normal or subnormal levels in the morning may suggest systemic juvenile arthritis.

Establish whether the parent has administered fever reduction measures, and if so, how recently. Ask whether the child has had recent surgery, been in contact with persons with infectious or communicable diseases, or been immunized recently. If the child is a young infant, ask whether the infant has been anorexic or irritable (more obvious signs of fever such as shivering and diaphoresis are not usually seen in the young infant). If the child is 5 years or older, assess the child's ability to understand and to follow directions because oral temperature measurement may be desirable. If rectal temperature measurement is selected, the procedure may be left until near the end of the health assessment because preschoolers, in particular, find it intrusive.

Guidelines for Measurement of Body Temperature

■ Select the site for temperature measurement based on the child's age and condition (Table 8-3), institutional policy, and what might be least traumatic for the child. The tympanic route, for example, has a high level of acceptability by children.

Table 8-3   Guidelines for Selection of Site for Body Temperature Measurement

Site	Age-Group	Special Considerations
Axilla	All age-groups, but particularly preschoolers, who tend to fear invasive procedures. May be used for children for whom the oral route is not possible and for those who would not tolerate the rectal route.	• Measures shell temperature. • May be taken using standard glass, electronic, digital, or axillary thermometry. • Although some sources recommend the monitor mode for electronic thermometers, some evidence also suggests that the predictive mode be used for full-term infants. • May be contraindicated when accuracy is especially critical or in the early stages of a fever when the axilla may not be sensitive to early changes.
Rectal	All age-groups. Some sources recommend use in children older than 2 years because of risks of breakage and perforation. Some evidence suggests that the rectal route is the most reliable route for measurement of temperature in infants and children, although others recommend its use only when no other route is appropriate (e.g., children who are too young or too agitated to cooperate or follow directions; children who have had oral or axillary surgery).	• Measures core temperature. • May be taken using standard glass, electronic, and Tempa-dot devices. • Do not use if child has had anal surgery, chemotherapy affecting the mucosa, has diarrhea or rectal irritation, or if it is possible to use oral or axillary sites. Presence of stool may decrease accuracy.

Route	Age	Comments
Oral	Cooperative 5- and 6-year-old children, school-aged children, and adolescents.	• Reflects shell temperature. • May be taken using standard glass, electronic, digital, and Tempa-dot thermometry. • Do not use if child is uncooperative or unable to follow directions, is comatose, seizure prone, has had oral surgery, mouth breathes, or is on oxygen. • Electronic thermometry produces acceptable results for the child who keeps mouth open during measurement.
Tympanic	All ages, although several sources suggest that the route is insufficiently sensitive and reliable for the detection of fever in children younger than 3 years old and even younger than 6 years.	• Considered to measure core temperature. • Easy to use, noninvasive, and quick for young children. • May be contraindicated in young children and infants because of their small ear canals. • In children 3 years and younger, pull the ear down and back during temperature measurement. • May be advisable to select another method if precise measurements are necessary or if clinical symptoms suggest fever in the presence of a normal or lower than expected tympanic measurement.
Skin	All ages	• Measured using plastic strip thermometer. • Variable accuracy. • May be used for screening and for at-home use.

▪ Position the child appropriately.

> For axillary temperature, hold the child quietly on your lap. Diversions, such as reading, are useful. Hold child's arm firmly against side.

> For oral temperature, have the child sit or lie quietly.

> For rectal temperature, younger infants can be placed in a supine position, with knees flexed toward the abdomen. Larger infants and children can be placed in prone or side-lying positions. If the parent is available, the child can wrap arms around the parent's neck and legs around the parent's waist or be placed prone across the parent's lap.

▪ Always record the route by which the temperature was taken because the differences between routes cannot be assumed as constant.

▪ In addition to measurement of body temperature, all children should be assessed for:

> Signs and symptoms of dehydration, including poor skin turgor, dry mucous membranes, decreased or absent tearing (in child older than 6 weeks of age), sunken eye orbits, dry body creases, and sunken fontanels (infants).

> Flushed appearance.

> Chills, as evidenced by shivering and piloerection.

> Restlessness.

> Lethargy.

> Skin mottling.

> Increased pulse and respiratory rates, and increased blood pressure.

> Twitching.

> Seizure activity.

> Young children may interpret "taking your temperature" as taking something away. Saying "let's see how warm you are" may avoid this interpretation.

Related Nursing Diagnoses

Anxiety: Related to febrile seizures; procedure

Risk for imbalanced body temperature: Related to infection; inflammation; stress; dehydration; tumor; immunization.

Risk for deficient fluid volume: Related to fever; increased metabolic rate; hyperpnea.

Deficient knowledge: Related to management of fever; measurement of fever; recognition of signs and symptoms of fever; management of seizures.

Hyperthermia: Related to heat stroke; ingestion of aspirin; metabolic disorders.

Hypothermia: Related to anesthesia; medications; near drowning; cold exposure.

Ineffective thermoregulation: Related to immaturity of body systems; genetic myopathy.

Measurement of Pulse
Rationale

The measurement of pulse is a routine part of hospital procedure but should not be underestimated as an easily accessible indicator of the status of the cardiovascular system. Disorders of the cardiovascular system, the effects of fever, and the effects of drug therapies can be monitored through assessment of pulse. The pulse should be routinely monitored during disease processes, during fever, before and after surgery, and whenever a child's condition deteriorates. A decreased pulse rate is more ominous than tachycardia in a young child following trauma.

Anatomy and Physiology

Approximately 8.5% of the body weight in the neonate is blood volume, compared with 7% to 7.5% in the older child and adult. The heart size increases as the child grows, with a resultant decrease in heart rate. Variations in heart rate are much more dramatic in the child than in the adult. Table 8-4 lists normal pulse

Table 8-4   Pulse Rates in Children at Rest

Age	Resting (Awake)	Resting (Asleep)	Exercise and Fever
Birth	100-180	80-160	Up to 220
1-3 mo	100-220	80-180	Up to 220
3 mo-2 yr	80-150	70-120	Up to 200
2 yr-10 yr	70-110	60-100	Up to 180
10 yr-adult	55-90	50-90	Up to 180

From Wong DL: *Whaley & Wong's nursing care of infants and children,* ed 5, St Louis, 1995, Mosby.

Table 8-5   Influences on Pulse Rate

Influence	Effect
Medications	Aminophylline, racemic epinephrine, atropine sulfate increase pulse rate. Digoxin decreases pulse rate.
Activity	Activity increases pulse rate. Sustained, regular exercise eventually decreases rate. Pulse varies if a child is sleeping, increasing during inspiration and decreasing during expiration (sinus arrhythmia). Crying and feeding increases pulse rate in an infant.
Fever	Increases pulse rate by about 10 to 15 beats per °C temperature increase. High fever accompanied by low pulse and respiratory rate may signal a drug reaction. Low fever with high pulse and respiratory rates may signal septic shock.
Apprehension, acute pain	Increases pulse rate.
Hemorrhage	Increases pulse rate.
Increased intracranial pressure	Decreases pulse rate.
Respiratory distress	Increased pulse rate in early distress; decreased rate in late distress.

rates; Table 8-5, influences on pulse rate; and Table 8-6, deviations from normal pulse patterns.

Preparation

Ask the parent or child about a family history of arrhythmias, atherosclerosis, or myocardial infarction. Ask if the child has known heart disease or has experienced or is experiencing palpitations or arrhythmias. Determine if fever or pain is present, and if the child has received medication recently.

Guidelines for Measurement of Pulse

■ Measure the pulse when the infant or child is quiet or preferably, asleep. Because of lability of the pulse, carefully document the child's activity or anxiety level when the pulse is recorded.

Table 8-6   Deviations from Normal Pulse Patterns

Pulse	Characteristics and Significance
Bradycardia	Slowed pulse rate.
Tachycardia	Increased pulse rate. In the absence of apprehension, crying, increased activity, or fever, tachycardia may indicate cardiac disease.
Sinus arrhythmia	Pulse rate increases during inspiration, decreases during expiration. Sinus arrhythmia is a normal variation in children, especially during sleep.
Alternating pulse (pulsus alternans)	Alteration of weak and strong beats. May indicate heart failure.
Bigeminal pulse	Coupled beats related to premature beats.
Paradoxical pulse	Strength of pulse diminishes with inspiration.
Thready pulse	Weak, rapid pulse. May be indicative of shock. Pulse is difficult to palpate; seems to appear and disappear.
Corrigan's pulse (water-hammer pulse)	Forceful, jerky beat caused by wide variation in pulse pressure.

- Select the appropriate site. The apical pulse is measured in children younger than 2 years of age because the radial pulse is difficult to locate. The apical pulse should be measured at any age when the radial pulse is difficult to locate, when cardiac disease has been identified, or when the radial pulse is irregular. Radial and femoral pulses should be compared at least once in the young child to detect circulatory impairment.
- Listen for the apical pulse at the point of maximum impulse (PMI). This will be found in the *fourth intercostal space* in children *younger than 7 years.* In children *older than 7 years* the apical pulse will be found in the *fifth interspace,* and will be more lateral.
- Auscultate radial and apical pulses for 1 full minute because of possible alterations in rhythm. If frequent apical pulses are required, use shorter counting times.
- Pulses may be graded (Table 8-7).

Table 8-7   Grading of Pulses

0	Not palpable.
+1	Thready, weak. Difficult to find. Easily obliterated.
+2	Difficult to find. Pressure may obliterate.
+3	Easy to find. Difficult to obliterate (normal).
+4	Bounding, strong. Cannot be obliterated.

Related Nursing Diagnoses

Anxiety: Related to pulse arrhythmias or irregularities.

Decreased cardiac output: Related to bradycardia; tachycardia; hypothermia or hyperthermia; surgery; medications; congenital heart defects; shock.

Risk for deficient fluid volume: Related to hemorrhage.

Ineffective tissue perfusion: Related to decreased cardiac output.

Measurement of Respirations

Rationale

Assessment of respiration involves external assessment of ventilation. Because the quality and rate of respirations can be affected by disorders in every body system, the character of respirations must be carefully assessed and reported.

Anatomy and Physiology

Infants and young children inhale a relatively small amount of air and exhale a relatively large amount of oxygen. Young children and infants have fewer alveoli and therefore less alveolar surface through which gas exchange can occur. These factors, together with a higher metabolic rate, are influential in increasing respiratory rates in infants and children. Table 8-8 outlines normal respiratory rates, and Table 8-9 outlines influences on respiratory rates.

Preparation

Ask the parent or child about the use of medications; whether there is difficulty breathing, or apnea (infants); and about the presence of respiratory infections. Inquire about a family history of cardiac or respiratory disorders.

Table 8-8   Variations in Respiration with Age

Age	Rate (breaths/min)
Premature infant	40-90
Neonate	30-80
1 yr	20-40
2 yr	20-30
3 yr	20-30
5 yr	20-25
10 yr	17-22
15 yr	15-20
20 yr	15-20

From Lowrey GN: *Growth and development of children,* ed 8, St Louis, 1986, Mosby.

Table 8-9   Influences on Respiration

Influencing Factor	Effect
Age	Respiratory rate decreases as the child grows older.
	The rate tends to increase dramatically in infants and young children relative to anxiety, crying, fever, disease.
	The rhythm is irregular in young infants, who experience sharp increases in rate and apneic spells. (Apneic spells of 15-20 seconds or longer are considered pathologic.)
Medications	Narcotic analgesics decrease respiratory rate. Xanthine derivatives may cause an increase in rate.
Position	Slumping impedes ventilatory movements.
Fever	Respirations increase in rate and depth.
Increased activity	Respirations increase in rate or depth.
Anxiety or fear	Respirations increase in rate and depth.
Pathologic states	Respiratory rate, rhythm, and depth alter as a result of cerebral trauma, respiratory disorders, hemorrhage, anemia, meningitis, cardiac disorders, infectious disorders, and tetanus.
Pain	Respiratory rate may decrease or increase.

Table 8-10 **Altered Respiratory Patterns**

Pattern	Description
Dyspnea	Difficult or labored breathing; indicated by presence of retractions.
Bradypnea	Abnormally slow rate of breathing; rhythm regular.
Tachypnea	Abnormally fast rate of breathing.
Hyperpnea	Rapid, deep respirations.
Apnea	Absence of respirations.
Cheyne-Stokes respiration (periodic breathing)	Periods of deep, rapid breathing alternating with periods of apnea. Commonly seen in infants, and may be seen normally in children during deep sleep. Abnormal causes include drug-induced depression and brain damage.
Kussmaul's respiration	Abnormally deep breathing. May be rapid, normal, or slow. Commonly associated with metabolic acidosis.
Biot's respiration (ataxic breathing)	Unpredictable, irregular breathing. Seen with lower brain damage and respiratory depression.

Guidelines for Measurement of Respirations

■ Assess the infant's or child's respirations before beginning more intrusive procedures. If the infant or child is already crying, wait for calmer behavior before assessing respiratory rates.

■ Avoid letting the child know that respirations are being counted;

self-consciousness may alter the respiratory rate and depth. Assess the respirations when counting the pulse or performing an assessment of the thorax and lungs. Table 8-10 gives a description of respiratory rhythms.

■ When assessing the respirations of *infants and younger children,* the nurse places fingers or a hand just below the child's xiphoid process so that the inspiratory rises can be felt. Alternatively, the respirations can be assessed by listening to breath sounds through the stethoscope. In infants, respirations can also be assessed by observing abdominal movements because respirations are diaphragmatic.

■ Observe a complete respiratory cycle (inspiration plus expiration).

Count respirations for *1 full minute.* Respirations of infants and young children can be quite irregular.

While counting, note the depth and rhythm of breathing. Depth is a subjective estimation and is usually noted as shallow, normal, or deep. If unable to label a rhythm, describe it.

■ Observe the child for:

Cyanosis of the nailbeds, hands, and feet, which may indicate *central* or *peripheral cyanosis.* Peripheral cyanosis may be caused by vasoconstriction, and is common in the young infant.

Cyanosis of the lips, oral mucosa, and generalized body cyanosis, are indicative of *central cyanosis.* Central cyanosis indicates a significant drop in the oxygen-carrying capacity of the blood.

Restlessness, anxiety, and decreasing levels of consciousness, which can be related to hypoxia.

Related Nursing Diagnoses

Activity intolerance: Related to inadequate oxygenation secondary to respiratory depression; ineffective respiratory effort.

Anxiety: Related to air hunger.

Ineffective breathing pattern: Related to obstruction; infection; medication; apnea; acidosis; brain damage.

Powerlessness: Related to inadequate oxygenation.

Blood Pressure

9

Rationale

Blood pressure readings provide significant information about the child's health status. Until recently, children younger than 3 years were commonly not screened for blood pressure because of the extra skill and patience required to obtain a blood pressure reading in such young patients. Most children with hypertension have renal disease; many fewer have coarctation of the aorta or pheochromocytoma. Screening of blood pressure in young children permits early detection of serious disorders and should be performed at least yearly on children from 3 years of age to adolescence. Blood pressure determination is routine on admission to health care facilities and in postoperative procedures. It should also be performed after invasive diagnostic procedures and before and after administration of drugs known to alter blood pressure. Blood pressure is taken whenever a child "feels funny" or when a child's condition deteriorates.

Anatomy and Physiology

Blood pressure is a product of cardiac output and increased peripheral resistance. In the neonate, systolic blood pressure is low, reflecting the weaker ability of the left ventricle. As the child grows, the size of the heart and of the left ventricle also increases, resulting in steadily increasing blood pressure values. At adolescence the heart enlarges abruptly, which also results in an increase in blood pressure values, comparable to those of the adult (Table 9-1).

An increase in cardiac output or in peripheral resistance will raise blood pressure. Decrease in cardiac output or in peripheral resistance will lower blood pressure. Overall maintenance of blood pressure reflects an intimate relationship among cardiac output,

Table 9-1   Normal Blood Pressure Values at Various Ages

Age	Systole/Diastole (mmHg) (Girls)	Systole/Diastole (mmHg) (Boys)
1mo	84/52	86/52
6mo	91/53	90/53
1 yr	91/54	90/56
2 yr	90/56	91/56
4 yr	92/56	93/56
6 yr	96/57	96/57
8 yr	99/59	99/60
10 yr	102/62	102/62
12 yr	107/66	107/64
14 yr	110/67	112/64
16 yr	112/67	117/67

Modified from Wong DL: *Whaley & Wong's nursing care of infants and children,* ed 5, St Louis, 1995, Mosby.

peripheral resistance, and blood volume, which can be influenced by several other factors (Table 9-2).

Equipment for Measuring Blood Pressure

■ Pediatric stethoscope
■ Sphygmomanometer with either a mercury or an aneroid manometer or electronic blood pressure devices (oscillometer; Doppler ultrasound)
■ Ace or tensor bandage (flush technique)

Preparation

Ask the parent or child about family history of hypertension or cardiac or kidney disease. Ask if the child has or has had headache, nose bleeds, swelling, or alterations in voiding patterns.

Guidelines for Measurement of Blood Pressure

■ Select appropriate method. Palpation rather than auscultation may be performed if the child has a narrow or deep brachial artery. The flush technique may be selected if it is impossible to obtain blood pressure readings in young children or infants by

Table 9-2   Influences on Blood Pressure

Influence	Effect
Medications	Narcotic analgesics, general anesthetics, diuretics decrease blood pressure.
	Aminophylline increases blood pressure.
Conditions	Blood pressure decreases during hemorrhage.
	Blood pressure increases with renal disease, increased intracranial pressure, coarctation of aorta (blood pressure in arms), pheochromocytoma, hyperthyroidism, diabetes mellitus, and acute pain.
	Pulse pressure widens with increased intracranial pressure.
Diurnal variation	Blood pressure usually is higher during morning and afternoon than during evening and night.
Apprehension and anxiety	Increases blood pressure.
Increased activity	Increases blood pressure.

other means. Oscillometric devices yield readings that correlate better with direct radial artery values than methods using auscultation and avoid problems associated with auscultation such as too rapid deflation of the cuff. Doppler ultrasound is accurate for systolic blood pressure but unreliable for diastolic pressure measurement. Limbs must be stabilized during measurement with oscillometric devices if accurate readings are to be obtained.

■ Select appropriate site (Figure 9-1). Extremities in casts, those in which intravenous fluids are being infused, or those that are traumatized should not be used. Thighs may be selected if only large cuffs are available.

■ Select appropriate cuff size. The cuff should cover at least 75% of the upper arm or thigh in children and adolescents (Table 9-3) leaving enough room to place the bell of the stethoscope at the antecubital fossa and to avoid obstruction of the axilla. An overly large cuff may produce low readings. A cuff that is too narrow may produce high readings. If a correctly fitting cuff is not available, a wider cuff may be used. (Wider cuffs do not create the low readings in infants and younger children that are

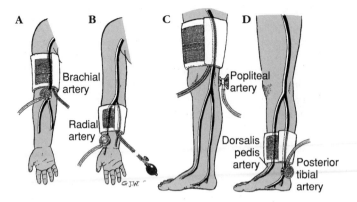

Figure 9-1
Sites for blood pressure measurement. **A,** Upper arm.
B, Lower arm or forearm. **C,** Thigh. **D,** Calf or ankle.
(From Wong DL et al: *Whaley & Wong's nursing care of infants and children,*
ed 6, St. Louis, 1999, Mosby.)

Table 9-3   Guidelines for Selecting Age-Appropriate Cuff Sizes

Age	Bladder Width (cm)	Bladder Length (cm)
Infant	5	8
Child	8	13
Adult	13	24

Modified from Frohlich ED et al: Recommendations for human blood pressure determination by sphygmomanometers: report of a special task force appointed by
the Steering Committee, American Heart Association, *Circulation* 77:501A, 1988.

produced in adults.) The cuff bladder should be long enough to
encircle the arm without overlapping.

In children who are overweight or who have thick arms,
measuring limb circumference may be a more accurate method for
determining cuff size. When considering limb circumference, the
cuff should be 40% to 50% of the limb circumference when
measuring at the upper arm, midway between the top of the
shoulder and the olecranon. Limb circumference guidelines should
be used when using an area other than the upper arms for blood
pressure measurement.

- Check bulb and pressure valve. Valve should adjust smoothly.
- Check needle of aneroid manometer. It should be at zero.
- Check mercury column of mercury-gravity manometer. It should be at zero.
- Blood pressure readings should be performed before other anxiety-producing procedures. The infant or child should be sitting quietly or lying down. The very young child may be most comfortable cradled in the parent's arms or lap.

Auscultation Method of Blood Pressure Measurement

Assessment	Findings
Select appropriate site and cuff. Position the child's limb. The arm should be at heart level. If positioned below the heart, falsely high reading may be obtained. If obtaining a thigh reading, the child may be positioned on the abdomen or with the knee slightly flexed. Expose the limb completely. Compression of the limb by rolled-up clothing may give a low reading. If the child is upset by removal of clothing, it is best to apply the cuff over the sleeve rather than rolling it up. Rolling produces a tight band.	
Palpate the brachial artery if using the arm, or the popliteal artery if using the thigh. Ensure that the cuff is fully deflated. Center the arrows on the cuff over the brachial artery of the arm, or position the bladder over the posterior aspect of the thigh. Position the manometer at eye level.	Viewing the manometer from above or below gives inaccurate readings.

Assessment	Findings
Palpate the radial or popliteal artery, and inflate the cuff to 20 mmHg above the point at which the pulse disappears.	
Deflate the cuff; wait 15 to 30 seconds.	Inadequate release of venous congestion gives falsely high readings.
Place the earpieces of the stethoscope in your ears. Earpieces should point forward to be inserted correctly. A pediatric stethoscope and bell should be used for infants and small children.	Incorrect placement of earpieces produces muffling or no sound at all.
Relocate the brachial or the popliteal artery. Place the bell or the diaphragm over the artery. Turn the valve of the pressure bulb clockwise until tight, and inflate cuff to 20 mmHg above the child's systolic reading.	Improper placement of the stethoscope produces low systolic and high diastolic readings.
Gradually release the valve to reduce pressure at a rate of 2 to 3 mmHg/sec.	Rapid release may cause inaccurate reading of the systolic pressure.
Observe the point at which the first clear reading (first Korotkoff sound) is obtained (systolic pressure) and at which the first muffling occurs (fourth Korotkoff sound) for the diastolic pressure in children younger than 13 years. Record the point at which all sound disappears (fifth Korotkoff sound) as the diastolic pressure in children 13 years and older.	In children younger than 1 year, thigh pressures should equal arm pressures; in children older than 1 year, thigh pressure is approximately 20 mmHg higher.
	Blood pressure will tend to be higher in children who are large for age than in children who are small.
	Korotkoff sounds may not be audible in early childhood because of a narrow or deeply placed artery.

Assessment	Findings
	Clinical Alert A thigh pressure reading that is the same or lower than upper arm readings in infants may indicate coarctation of the aorta.
Deflate the cuff rapidly once readings have been obtained. Wait 30 seconds before obtaining further readings.	**Clinical Alert** Repeat blood pressure readings if lower or higher than expected.
Record limb, position, cuff size, and how reading was obtained.	Document and report persistently elevated or lowered blood pressure readings. Consistently elevated serial readings may indicate hypertension. Persistently low diastolic pressure may indicate a patent ductus arteriosus. *Pulse pressure* (difference between systolic and diastolic pressures) of more than 50 mmHg may indicate congestive heart failure. Pulse pressure of less than 10 mmHg may indicate aortic stenosis.

Palpation Method of Blood Pressure Measurement

Assessment	Findings
Select appropriate site and cuff. Position child's limb, and prepare the cuff as though determining blood pressure by auscultation method.	
Palpate the brachial or the radial artery (arm) or the popliteal artery (thigh), and inflate the cuff 20 mmHg above point at which pulse disappears.	

Assessment	Findings
Slowly deflate the cuff, at a rate of 2 to 3 mmHg/sec.	
Determine point at which the pulse is first felt. This is the *systolic* pressure. The diastolic pressure cannot be determined by this method.	The systolic pressure obtained by radial palpation is approximately 10 mmHg lower than arm pressure.

Flush Method of Blood Pressure Measurement

Assessment	Findings
Wrap cuff around the limb. Elevate the limb. Wrap an elastic bandage from the fingers toward the antecubital space (or from the toes toward the knee).	
Inflate the cuff above the expected systolic pressure.	
Remove bandage. Place the child's arm at his or her side.	The limb will appear pale.
Slowly deflate the cuff until color suddenly returns. The reading is taken when color appears.	The value (flush pressure) obtained is the mean blood pressure (average of the diastolic and systolic pressures).

Related Nursing Diagnoses

Decreased cardiac output: Related to arrhythmias; congenital anomalies; medications.

Deficient fluid volume: Related to hemorrhage.

Ineffective tissue perfusion: Related to hypotension.

ASSESSMENT
OF BODY
SYSTEMS

III

Integument

10

Assessment of the integument involves inspection and palpation of skin, nails, hair, and scalp and may be combined with assessment of other areas of the body.

Rationale

Assessment of the integument, or skin, should be an integral part of every health assessment, regardless of setting or situation. Many common pathophysiologic disorders have associated integumentary disorders. For example, many contagious childhood diseases have associated characteristic rashes. Rashes of all sorts are common in childhood. The integument yields much information about the physical care that a child receives and about the nutritional, circulatory, and hydration status of the child, which is valuable in planning health teaching interventions.

Anatomy and Physiology

The skin, which begins to develop during the eleventh week of gestation, consists of three layers (Figure 10-1). The *epidermis* is the outermost layer and is further divided into four layers. The top layer, or horny layer (stratum corneum), is of primary importance in protecting the internal homeostasis of the body. Melanin, produced by the regeneration layer of the epidermis, is the main pigment of the skin. The *dermis* underlies the epidermis and contains blood vessels, lymphatic vessels, hair follicles, and nerves. *Subcutaneous tissue* underlies the dermis and helps cushion, contour, and insulate the body. This final layer contains sweat and sebaceous glands. The sebaceous glands produce sebum, which may have some bactericidal effect.

The skin has four main functions: protection against injury, thermoregulation, impermeability, and sensor of touch, pain, heat, and cold.

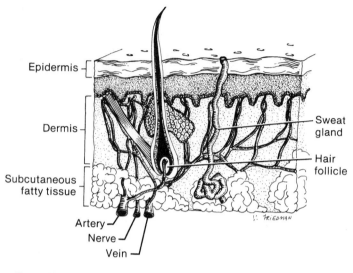

Figure 10-1
Normal skin layers.
(From Potter PA: *Pocket guide to health assessment,* ed 4, St. Louis, 1998, Mosby.)

The normal pH of the skin is acidic, which is thought to protect the skin from bacterial invasion. In infants the pH of the skin is higher, the skin is thinner, and the secretion of sweat and sebum is minimal. As a result, infants are more prone to skin infections and conditions than older children and adults. Further, because of loose attachment between the dermis and epidermis, infants and children tend to blister easily.

Preparation

Inquire about a family history of skin disorders, the life-style of the family, and recent changes in life-style. Ask when lesions began and whether other symptoms accompanied the lesions. Ask the parent to describe the size, configuration, distribution, type, and color of the lesions.

A well-illuminated room with white walls is essential for proper visualization of the skin. (Yellow walls may give the appearance of jaundice and blue walls the appearance of cyanosis.) The room should also be warm.

Assessment of Skin

Assessment of the skin is usually performed during assessment of each body system.

Assessment	Findings
Observe the skin for odor.	**Clinical Alert** The presence of odor may indicate poor hygiene or infection.
Observe the color and pigmentation of the skin. If a color change is suspected, carefully inspect the areas of the body where there is less melanin (nailbeds, earlobes, sclerae, conjunctivae, lips, mouth). Inspect the abdomen (an area less exposed to sunlight) and the trunk. Use natural daylight for assessment if *jaundice* is suspected. Pressing a glass slide against a skin area produces blanching, which supplies contrast and enables closer assessment of the presence of jaundice. If a child has a different pigmentation from that of the accompanying parent, ask about the absent parent for hereditary trait recognition.	Overall skin color normally varies between and within races. For example, black children normally have a bluish tinge to gums, tongue borders, and nailbeds. Some children of Mediterranean origin may have a bluish tinge to their lips. The skin of Asian children normally has a yellow tone. **Clinical Alert** A brown color to the skin may indicate Addison's disease or some pituitary tumors. A reddish blue skin tone suggests polycythemia in light-skinned children. Red skin color may result from exposure to cold, hyperthermia, blushing, alcohol, or inflammation (if localized). Blue (cyanosis) coloration of nails, soles, and palms may indicate *peripheral* or *central* cyanosis. Peripheral cyanosis may arise from anxiety or cold; central cyanosis is indicative of a marked drop in the oxygen-carrying capacity of the blood and is best identified in the lips, tongue, and oral mucosa. Generalized

Assessment	Findings
	body cyanosis may be evident in central cyanosis. Black-skinned children may appear ashen-gray with cyanosis.

Yellow skin color may indicate jaundice (which accompanies liver disease, hepatitis, red cell hemolysis, biliary obstruction, or severe infection in infants) and is best observed in the sclerae, the mucous membranes, fingernails, soles, palms, and on the abdomen.

Yellowing of the palms, soles, and face (and not of the sclerae or mucous membranes) may indicate carotenemia, produced from ingestion of carrots, squash, and sweet potatoes.

Yellowing of the exposed skin areas (and not of the sclerae and mucous membranes) may indicate chronic renal disease.

Bruising in soft tissue areas (for example, buttocks) rather than on shins, knees, or elbows may indicate child abuse or cultural practices such as spooning that are used to heal.

A generalized lack of color involving the skin, hair, and eyes indicates albinism.

Pallor (lack of pink tones in whites; ash gray color in blacks), suggestive of syncope, fever, shock, edema, or anemia, is best observed in the face, mouth, conjunctivae, and nails.

Assessment	Findings
Observe the moistness of exposed skin ureas and mucous membranes. Lightly stroke body creases. Compare body creases, one to another.	The skin is normally slightly dry. Exposed areas normally feel dryer than body creases. Mucous membranes should be moist. **Clinical Alert** Dry skin on the lips, hands, or genitalia suggests contact dermatitis. Generalized dryness, accompanied by moist body creases and moist mucous membranes, indicates overexposure to the sun, overbathing, or poor nutrition. Dry arm creases and mucous membranes suggest dehydration. Clamminess may indicate shock or perspiration.
Palpate the skin with the back of the hand to determine *temperature*. Compare each side of the body with the other, and the upper with the lower extremities.	**Clinical Alert** Generalized hyperthermia may indicate fever, sunburn, or a brain disorder. Localized hyperthermia may indicate burn or infection. Generalized hypothermia may indicate shock. Local hypothermia may result from exposure to cold.
Inspect and palpate the texture of the skin. Note the presence of scars and excessive scar tissue (keloid).	An infant's or child's skin is normally smooth and even. **Clinical Alert** Rough, dry skin may indicate overbathing, poor nutrition, exposure to weather, or an endocrine disorder and is associated with Down syndrome. Flaking or scaling between the fingers or toes may be related to eczema, dermatitis, or a fungal infection.

Assessment	Findings
	Thin, dry, wrinkled skin may indicate ectodermal hypoplasia.
	Oily scales on the scalp indicate seborrheic dermatitis (cradle cap).
	Hypopigmented, scaly patches on the face and upper body, or scattered papules (Table 10-1) over the arms, thighs, and buttocks, and fine, superficial scales may indicate eczema.
	Moist, warm, flushed skin occurs with hyperthyroidism.
	A crackling sensation on palpation may indicate subcutaneous emphysema.
Palpate for *turgor* by grasping a fold on the upper arm or abdomen between the fingers and quickly releasing. Note the ease with which the skin moves (mobility) and returns to place (turgor) without residual marks.	Skin normally returns quickly to place with no residual marks. **Clinical Alert** A skinfold that returns slowly to place or retains marks commonly indicates dehydration or malnutrition. Other possible causes are chronic disease and muscle disorders.
Palpate for *edema* by pressing a thumb into areas that look swollen.	**Clinical Alert** Thumb indentations that remain after the thumb is removed indicate pitting edema. Edema in the periorbital areas may indicate crying, allergies, recent sleep, renal disease, or juvenile hypothyroidism. Edema (dependent) of the lower extremities and buttocks may indicate renal or cardiac disorders.
Inspect and palpate the skin for *lesions* (see Table 10-1). Note the distribution, shape, color, size, and consistency of the lesions and birthmarks (Table 10-3).	**Clinical Alert** Rashes are associated with several childhood disorders (Table 10-2). *Text continued on p. 112*

Text continued on p. 112

Table 10-1   Common Skin Lesions

Lesion	Description
Primary Lesions (arise from normal skin)	
Macule	Small (less than 1 cm or 0.4 in) flat mass; differs from surrounding skin. Example: freckle.
Papule	Small (less than 1 cm or 0.4 in), raised, solid mass. Example: small nevus.
Nodule	Solid, raised mass; slightly larger (1-2 cm or 0.4-0.8 in) and deeper than a papule.
Tumor	Solid, raised mass; larger than a nodule; may be hard or soft.
Wheal	Irregularly shaped, transient area of skin edema. Example: hive, insect bite, allergic reaction.
Vesicle	Small (less than 1 cm or 0.4 in) raised, fluid-filled mass. Example: herpes simplex, varicella.

Continued

Table 10-1   Common Skin Lesions—cont'd

Lesion	Description
Bulla	Raised fluid-filled mass; larger than a vesicle. Example: second-degree burn.
Pustule	Vesicle containing purulent exudate. Example: acne, impetigo, staphylococcal infections.

Secondary Lesions (arise from changes in primary lesions)

Scale	Thin flake of exfoliated epidermis. Example: psoriasis, dandruff.
Crust	Dried residue of serum, blood, or purulent exudate. Example: eczema.
Erosion	Moist lesion resulting from loss of superficial epidermis. Example: rupture of lesion in varicella.
Ulcer	Deep loss of skin surface; may extend to dermis and subcutaneous tissue. Example: syphilitic chancre, decubitus ulcer.

Table 10-1   Common Skin Lesions—cont'd

Lesion	Description
Fissure	Deep, linear crack in skin. Example: athlete's foot.
Lichenification	Thickened skin with accentuated skin furrows. Example: sequela of eczema.
Striae	Thin white or purple stripes, commonly found on abdomen. May result from pregnancy or weight gain.
Purpuric Lesions	
Petechia	Flat, round, deep red or purplish mass (less than 3 mm or 0.1 in).
Ecchymosis	Mass of variable size and shape; initially purplish, fading to green, yellow, then brown.

Table 10-2   Distribution and Characteristics of Lesions Associated with Common Childhood Disorders

Disorder	Accompanying Lesions
Allergic Disorders	
Allergic reaction	Almost any type of lesion possible. Common manifestations are urticaria (hives), eczema, and contact dermatitis. Lesions may be intensely pruritic.
Urticaria	Wheals may be small or large, discrete or confluent, sparse or profuse. Wheals tend to come in crops, and fade in a few hours.
Eczema (atopic dermatitis)	Acute: erythema, vesicles, exudate, and crusts. Chronic: pruritic, dry, scaly, and thickened rash. Infantile form found on cheeks, forehead, scalp, and extensor surfaces. Childhood form found on wrists, ankles, and flexor surfaces.
Contact dermatitis	Pruritic red swelling that may be well demarcated from normal skin. Papules and bullae may be present.
Contagious Diseases	
Molluscum contagiosum	Sharply circumscribed or multiple pearly umbilicated papules located on any area of the body.
Mumps	Painful swelling of parotid glands. May be unilateral or bilateral.
Measles (rubeola)	Red maculopapular rash that begins on face. Confluent at early sites of involvement, discrete at later sites. Becomes brownish in 3-4 days and desquamates.
Rubella (German measles)	Pinkish red maculopapular rash that begins on face and spreads downward. Discrete lesions. Rash disappears within 3 days.
Roseola (baby measles)	Rose-pink macules or maculopapules that appear first on trunk before spreading. Discrete lesions fade on pressure. Nonpruritic. Rash disappears in 1-2 days.
Chickenpox (varicella zoster)	Rash progresses from macule to papule to vesicle to crust. Pruritic. Begins on trunk and spreads primarily to face and proximal extremities.

Table 10-2   Distribution and Characteristics of Lesions
Associated with Common Childhood Disorders—cont'd

Disorder	Accompanying Lesions
Contagious Diseases—cont'd	
Scarlet fever	Tiny red lesions involve all but the face; more intense in joint areas. Desquamation begins in 1 week. Tongue initially is white and swollen (first 1-2 days), then becomes red and swollen.
Bacterial Infections	
Impetigo contagiosa	Rash begins with reddish macule, then vesicle appears. Vesicle ruptures, producing a moist erosion. Exudate dries, producing a honey-colored crust. Pruritic.
Cellutis	Skin red, swollen, warm to touch, firmly infiltrated. "Streaking" may be present.
Viral Infections	
Herpes simplex (cold sore)	Grouped vesicles on an erythematous base, found near lips, nose, genitalia, buttocks. Vesicles dry, leaving a crust.
Herpes zoster (shingles)	Rash follows dermatome of affected nerve, and appears in crops of vesicles. Pain and itching are common.
Fungi	
Candidiasis	Eruptions have sharp borders and include red papules, pustules, and satellite lesions. Commonly occur in skin creases and may be associated with oral thrush.
Tinea capitis	Pruritic circumscribed areas of scaling on the scalp. Alopecia present.
Tinea corporis	Pruritic red, round, or oval scaly areas. Central area clear.
Tinea pedis (athlete's foot)	Maceration and fissuring between toes or vesicles on plantar surface. Pruritic.

Continued

Table 10-2 Distribution and Characteristics of Lesions Associated with Common Childhood Disorders—cont'd

Disorder	Accompanying Lesions
Infestations	
Scabies	Linear, brownish gray burrows are produced by the female mite. Sarcoptic infestations produce papules, pustules, vesicles, and hives. In infants, lesions are primarily found on face, palms, and soles. In children, lesions are commonly found on apposed surfaces of skin and inter-digital areas, on the extensor surfaces of joints and wrists, lower back, abdomen, genitalia, and buttocks.
Pediculosis corporis (body lice)	Lesions appear as red macules, wheals, excoriated papules, on the back and on areas that have close contact with clothing. Pruritic.
Lyme disease	Erythema chronicum migrans (ECM) appears 4-20 days after bite by a tick. Presents as a red macule or papule at the bite site and may be painless and nonitchy or warm, tender, and stinging. If untreated, ECM may have central clearing and may progress to ulceration. ECM commonly found on groin, axilla, and/or proximal thigh.
Miscellaneous	
Psoriasis	Thick, dry, red lesions covered with silvery scales. Lesions appear on scalp, ears, forehead, eyebrows, trunk, elbows, knees, and genitalia. More common in children 5 years of age and older.
Seborrheic dermatitis (cradle cap)	Oily, scaly patches on the scalp or along the hairline.
Henoch-Schönlein purpura (HSP)	Systemic purpura primarily involving buttocks and lower extremities. Maculopapular lesions, erythema, and urticaria may also be present.

Table 10-2   Distribution and Characteristics of Lesions
Associated with Common Childhood Disorders—cont'd

Disorder	Accompanying Lesions
Miscellaneous—cont'd	
Acne vulgaris	Lesions that appear on the face, neck, shoulders, upper chest, and back in about 85% of adolescents. Lesions may be noninflamed (comedomes) or inflamed. Comedomes may be closed and are compact masses (commonly called *whiteheads*). Open comedomes, or blackheads, have visible openings that are discolored through exposure of fatty acids to air. Inflamed lesions may lead to scarring and appear as papules, pustules, nodules, and cysts.

Table 10-3   Birthmarks and Their Description

Birthmark	Description
Vascular Nevi	
Salmon patch ("stork beak" mark)	Common. Flat, light pink mark found on the eyelids, in nasolabial region, or at the nape of the neck. Most disappear by the end of the first year of life.
Nevus flammeus (port-wine stain)	Flat, deep red or purplish red patches. Enlarge as child grows.
Strawberry nevus (raised hemangioma)	Begins as circumscribed grayish-white area; becomes red, raised, well defined. May not be present at birth; resolves spontaneously by 9 years of age.
Hyperpigmented Nevi	
Mongolian spot	Large, flat, blue, black, or slate colored area found on the buttocks and in the lumbosacral region.

Assessment	Findings
	Petechiae and ecchymoses may indicate a bleeding tendency.
Enquire about pruritus.	**Clinical Alert**
	Itching may indicate the onset of an asthmatic attack or may occur with hepatitis A or renal disorders or with some skin disorders.

Assessment of Nails

Assessment	Findings
Inspect nails for color, shape, and condition.	**Clinical Alert**
	Clubbing may indicate chronic respiratory or cardiac disease.
	Convex or concave curving nails may be hereditary or related to injury, iron deficiency, or infection.
Inspect nails for nail biting, skin picking, infection.	

Assessment of Hair

Assessment	Findings
Assess hair for distribution, color, texture, amount, and quality. Hair distribution is useful in estimating sexual maturity.	Hair normally covers all but the palms, soles, inner labial surfaces (girls), and prepuce and glans penis (boys).
Assess hair for dandruff and nits. If nits are suspected, use a fine-toothed metal or electronic comb on the hair to differentiate between nits, dandruff, and lint.	Scalp hair is normally shiny, silky, strong.
	Clinical Alert
	Dry, brittle, or depigmented hair may indicate nutritional deficiency or thyroid disorder.
	A hairline that extends to mid-forehead may be normal or may indicate cretinism.

Assessment	Findings
	Delayed or absent hair growth may indicate an ectodermal dysplasia.
	Unusually fine hair that is unable to hold a wave may indicate hyperthyroidism.
	Alopecia (loss of hair) may be related to tinea capitis, hair pulling, abuse, or persistent positioning on one side.
	Hair tufts on the spine or buttocks may indicate spina bifida.
	White eggs that are firmly attached to hair shafts indicate head lice. Dandruff can be removed.

Related Nursing Diagnoses

Impaired comfort: Related to pruritus; loss of skin surface.

Hyperthermia: Secondary to infection.

Deficient knowledge: Related to hygienic needs; prevention of infection; prevention of scarring.

Risk for infection: Related to loss of skin integrity.

Impaired oral mucous membrane: Secondary to infection; dehydration.

Impaired parenting: Related to inappropriate caretaking behaviors.

Chronic low self-esteem: Secondary to presence of acne, birthmarks, scarring.

Impaired skin integrity: Related to injury, infection, nutritional disorders.

Impaired tissue integrity: Related to injury; infection; altered nutritional state; altered pigmentation; developmental factors; alterations in turgor.

Head and Neck

11

Assessment of the neck includes evaluation of the trachea and the thyroid gland. The head is assessed for size, shape, and symmetry. The fontanels and sutures are examined, and head control is noted. Proceeding downward from the head to the neck provides a smooth progression of assessment.

Rationale

Examination of the head and neck is important in screening pediatric clients for acute disorders and long-term disabilities. The determination of disorders such as skull asymmetry can also signal the need for parent teaching.

Anatomy and Physiology

The head accounts for one fourth of the body length and one third of the body weight in the newborn infant, in comparison with one eighth of the body length and one tenth of the body weight in the adult. Head size, which is 32 to 38 cm (12.5 to 14 in) at birth, normally exceeds chest circumference by 1 to 2 cm (0.4 to 0.8 in) until 18 months of age. After 18 months, chest growth exceeds head size by 5 to 7 cm (2 to 2.75 in) (see Appendix B for charts of head circumference norms). The newborn skull consists of separate bones that fuse when brain growth is complete. Soft, fibrous tissue joints, called *sutures,* separate the bones (Figure 11-1). These sutures, which can be felt as prominent ridges, begin to unite by 6 months of age, but may be separated by increased intracranial pressure until 12 years of age.

Fontanels are formed by the juncture of three or more skull bones (see Figure 11-1) and are felt as soft concavities. Normally only the posterior and anterior fontanels can be palpated. The posterior fontanel may be closed at birth, and should always be

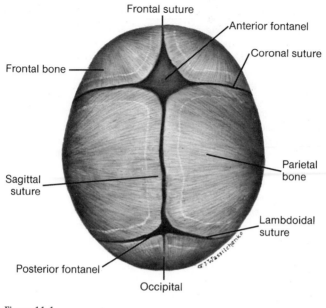

Figure 11-1
Location of sutures and fontanels.
(From Wong DL et al: *Whaley & Wong's nursing care of infants and children,*
ed 6, St. Louis, 1999, Mosby.)

closed by the second month. The anterior fontanel closes between
9 and 26 months of age; 90% close between 7 and 19 months.

By 4 months of age the infant should be able to hold the head
erect and in midline. By 6 months no significant head lag should
be noted when the child is pulled to a sitting position.

The neck in the infant and toddler is short, but by 4 years of
age it assumes adult proportions. Although the thyroid gland is
fully active at birth, it may not be palpable in infants and young
children.

Equipment for Measurement
of Head Circumference

Paper or narrow flexible metal tape (not cloth tape, because it may
stretch.)

Measurement	Findings
Measure head circumference if the child is 2 years of age or younger or if the size of child's head warrants concern. Place the tape around the head at points just above the eyebrows and the pinna and around the occipital prominence (Figure 11-2). If head circumference is measured daily, the head should be marked at key points to ensure consistency of measurement.	**Clinical Alert** If an infant's head circumference is above or below growth norms or the infant's established percentile, further evaluation is indicated. An abnormally large head circumference may indicate hydrocephalus or brain tumor. A small head circumference may indicate craniostenosis or microcephaly. Infants born to mothers who use cocaine or alcohol may have smaller head circumferences.

Preparation

Sit or lie the child in a comfortable position. The infant or young child may be most at ease on the parent's lap.

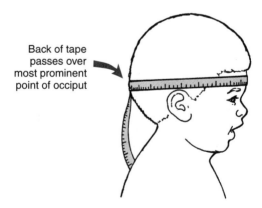

Back of tape passes over most prominent point of occiput

Figure 11-2
Measurement of head circumference.

Assessment of Head

Assessment	Findings
Observe the shape and symmetry of the infant's head from different angles. If possible, also note the shape and symmetry of the parents' heads.	Minor asymmetry in infants younger than 4 months is common and is related to molding. A head may be longer, narrower, or flatter than expected, as a result of genetic influences.
	Clinical Alert
	A markedly flattened occiput may be the result of persistent placement of the child in the supine position. If flattening is observed, ask the parents about the child's preferred sleep or play position. Parent teaching may be indicated. A flattened occiput and a small, rounded head is found with Down syndrome.
	Head asymmetry may reflect premature closure of suture lines and requires further evaluation.
Palpate the suture lines in infants.	Sutures are felt as prominent ridges. In a newborn infant the suture lines override as a result of molding, but usually flatten by 6 months.
	Palpation of the suture lines may occasionally lead to slight give in the underlying bone due to osteoporosis of the outer table of bone. This is known as *craniotabes*. Craniotabes is sometimes found in normal infants.
	Clinical Alert
	A separated sagittal suture is one of the most common findings in Down syndrome.

Assessment	Findings
	Craniotabes may suggest increased intracranial pressure as in hydrocephaly; infection as in syphylis; and metabolic disturbances such as rickets.
Observe and palpate the fontanels, if open, while the infant is sitting.	The anterior fontanel should be soft, flat, and pulsatile. The fontanel bulges slightly when the infant is crying.
	Clinical Alert
	A bulging fontanel may indicate increased intracranial pressure and is found in conditions such as head injury, meningitis, or neoplasm.
	A depressed fontanel may indicate dehydration.
	An enlarged anterior fontanel may indicate Down syndrome.
	An enlarged posterior fontanel may suggest congenital hypothyroidism.
Measure the width and length of an open anterior fontanel.	Until 9 to 12 months the anterior fontanel measures from 1 to 5 cm (0.4 to 2 in) in length and width.
	Clinical Alert
	An abnormally small or large fontanel may suggest a bone growth disorder.
Percuss the parietal bone on each side by tapping the index finger against the surface.	Percussion produces a "cracked pot" sound (Macewen's sign) in normal infants before closure of sutures.
	Clinical Alert
	Presence of Macewen's sign in older infants and children may indicate separation of sutures due to increased intracranial pressure as a result of conditions such as lead encephalopathy and brain tumor.

Related Nursing Diagnoses

Impaired comfort: Pain related to increased intracranial pressure; premature closure of fontanels; premature closure of suture lines.

Compromised family coping: Related to physical disabilities; mental disabilities secondary to congenital defects, altered brain pressures, or alcohol effects.

Interrupted family processes: Related to nature of the condition; uncertain future.

Fear or anxiety: Related to implications of the condition; uncertain future.

Deficient fluid volume: Related to nausea and vomiting; difficulty in swallowing.

Delayed growth and development: Related to physical disabilities; mental disabilities.

Deficient knowledge: Related to positioning; head hygiene and open fontanels.

Impaired physical mobility: Related to sensorimotor impairment.

Self-care deficit: Related to inability or difficulty in performing age-appropriate activities of daily living; secondary to sensorimotor impairment.

Low self-esteem: Related to physical deformity; interruption or failure in achieving developmental tasks.

Assessment of Neck

Assessment	Findings
Pull the infant to a sitting position while observing head control.	The infant younger than 4 months may show some head lag when pulled to a sitting position.
	Clinical Alert
	Significant head lag after 6 months may indicate cerebral palsy.
Put the child's head and neck through a full range of motion. The older child may be asked to look up, down, and sideways.	The child should exhibit no pain or limitation of movement in any direction.
	Clinical Alert
	Pain and resistance to flexion may indicate meningeal irritation.

Assessment	Findings
	Lateral resistance to motion may indicate torticollis as a result of injury to the sterno-cleidomastoid muscle.
Inspect the neck for lymph nodes, masses, cysts, webbing, extra folds of skin, and vein distention.	**Clinical Alert**
	Webbing and extra neck folds may indicate Turner's syndrome.
	Excessive and lax skin is found in children with Down syndrome.
	Small, round, firm swelling felt at midline just above the thyroid cartilage in a young infant suggests a thyroglossal duct cyst.
	Cervical lymphadenopathy may suggest viral or bacterial infections. General lymphadenopathy is associated with HIV infection in infants and with infectious mononucleosis in older children and adolescents. Bilateral tonsillar lymph node enlargement may indicate acute tonsillitis.
	Parotid swelling and tenderness may indicate mumps, bacterial infection, or presence of a stone.
	Enlarged occipital nodes may indicate rubella or roseola infantum.
	Vein distention may be present with labored respirations.
Palpate the trachea by placing the thumb on one of the trachea and the index finger on the other. Slide the fingers up and down while the child's neck is slightly hyperextended.	The trachea should be at midline or slightly to the right.
	Clinical Alert
	Any shift in the position of the trachea should be noted, as serious lung problems may be present.

Assessment	Findings
Palpate the thyroid gland by standing behind the child and placing your fingers or hands gently over the area of the gland (at the base the neck). The gland rises as a mass as the child swallows. Palpation of the thyroid gland in the infant and young child is difficult because of the shortness of the neck. Infants are best examined while lying supine across a parent's lap.	In normal children the thyroid gland may not be felt. **Clinical Alert** An enlarged thyroid gland may indicate goiter, lymphatic thyroiditis.

Related Nursing Diagnoses

Impaired comfort: Pain secondary to infection; meningeal irritation.

Compromised family coping: Related to situational crisis.

Fear: Related to rapid onset of illness.

Hyperthermia: Related to altered metabolic rates secondary to altered thyroid function.

Hypothermia: Related to altered metabolic rates secondary to altered thyroid function.

Impaired physical mobility: Related to neuromuscular deficits.

Self-care deficit: Related to inability or interruption in performing age-appropriate activities of daily living.

Impaired swallowing: Secondary to enlarged thyroid gland; altered level of consciousness; infection; alcohol exposure.

Ears

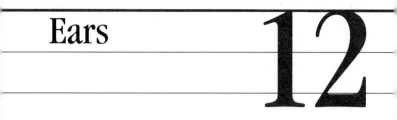

Assessment of the ears involves inspection of the external and internal ear, testing of hearing acuity, and otoscopic examination. The nurse also focuses on the child's health history in an effort to identify factors that could place the child at risk for hearing problems.

Rationale

Ear disorders are disruptive to language, speech, and social development. Early screening and detection can assist in minimizing or eliminating hearing deficiencies and their effects. Temporary and correctable conditions such as otitis media are common in young children but may go undetected. Abnormalities of the external ear can be important in alerting health professionals to the presence of syndromes and should be reported. Assessment of the ear is performed in conjunction with the eye examination, because eye problems are nearly twice as common in children with hearing deficiencies.

Anatomy and Physiology

The ear consists of the external ear, the middle ear, and the inner ear. The outer ear consists of the auricle, the cartilaginous shell, and the external ear canal. In children younger than 3 years the canal points upward; in older children it is directed downward and forward. The lining of the external ear canal secretes cerumen, which protects the ear.

The middle ear consists of the tympanum (eardrum) and three bones (ossicles) that touch the tympanum on one side and the membrane covering the opening to the inner ear on the other side. Vibrations of the tympanum are transmitted through the ossicles to the inner ear. The middle ear also contains an opening to the eustachian tube. The eustachian tube allows secretions to pass from the middle ear to the nasopharynx and enables air to enter the middle ear from the throat. Equalization of air pressure between the external ear canal and middle ear is essential for proper functioning of the tympanic membrane. The shorter and less angled eustachian tube in infants and young children permits secretions from the nose and throat to readily enter the middle ear, predisposing this age-group to more frequent ear infections.

The inner ear contains auditory nerve endings, which pick up sound waves from the middle ear and transmit them along the eighth cranial nerve, or auditory nerve, to the brain. Sound waves that contact the skull directly can also be picked up by the inner ear. The inner ear contains the structures for balance and for hearing.

The three divisions of the ear develop in the embryo at the same time as other vital organs are developing, which is why deformities of the ears can provide clues to developmental aberrations elsewhere in the body. External ear development begins at about the fifth week of gestation, and middle ear development begins at around the sixth week. The ears are particularly vulnerable to developmental aberration in the ninth week of gestation.

Neonates are capable of sound discrimination at birth and respond more readily to high-pitched voices. The presence of mucus in the eustachian tube may limit hearing when the neonate is first born but clears shortly after birth. Vernix caseosa in the external ear canal may make visualization of the tympanic membrane difficult.

The young infant responds to loud noises with the startle reflex, blinking, or cessation of movement. Infants 6 months of age or older attempt to locate the source of the sound.

Equipment for Ear Assessment

Tuning fork
Otoscope
Ear speculum
Bell

Preparation

Ask parents about a family history of hearing problems, maternal infections during pregnancy, problems during labor and delivery, and neonatal jaundice. Ask if the child has had convulsions, unexplained fever, drainage from the ear, mumps, measles, ear and respiratory tract infections, surgery to the ear, head injury, prolonged use of ototoxic drugs, and whether the child listens to loud music. Inquire about the use of hearing aids.

Inquire about when the child began speaking and whether there are any current concerns, such as inattentiveness to parental requests.

If an otoscopic examination is to be performed in a young child or infant, it is safer to restrain him or her. Explain and demonstrate to the parent how the child is to be held. The child can be placed on the side or abdomen, with the hands at the side and the head turned so that the ear to be examined points toward the ceiling. The parent can assist by placing one hand on the child's head above the ear and the other on the child's trunk. Alternatively, the child can sit on the parent's lap with one arm tucked behind the parent's back. The parent holds the child's head against his or her shoulder and the child's other, free arm (Figure 12-1).

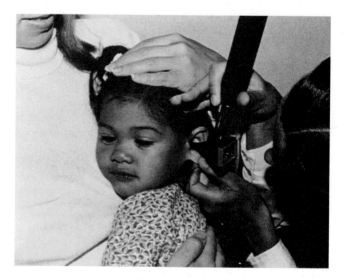

Figure 12-1
Position for restraining infant or child during otoscopic examination.
(From Whaley LF, Wong DL: *Nursing care of infants and children*, ed 4, St. Louis, 1991, Mosby.)

Assessment of External Ear

Assessment	Findings
Examine the ear for placement and position.	The top of the ear should cross an imaginary line from the inner eye to the occiput. The pinna should deviate no more than 10 degrees from a line perpendicular to the horizontal line. (Use of a pen or tongue blade can provide more concrete estimations of where the ear is positioned in relation to a vertical line.) Figure 12-2 illustrates normal placement and position of the ear.
	Clinical Alert
	Low or obliquely set ears are sometimes seen in children

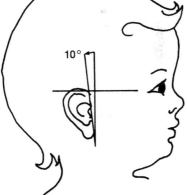

Figure 12-2
Ear placement and position.
(From Whaley LF, Wong DL: *Nursing care of infants and children,* ed 4, St. Louis, 1991, Mosby.)

Assessment	Findings
	with genitourinary or chromosomal abnormalities and in many syndromes.
Observe the ears for protrusion or flattening.	The ears of neonates are flat against the head.
	Clinical Alert
	Flattened ears in older infants may suggest persistent sidelying.
	Protruding ears may indicate swelling related to insect bites or to conditions such as mastoiditis.
Inspect the external ear for unusual structure and markings. Figure 12-3 illustrates usual markings.	Markings and structure of the external ear vary little from child to child. Variations may be normal but should be recorded. For example, a small skin tag on the tragus is a remnant of embryonic devel-

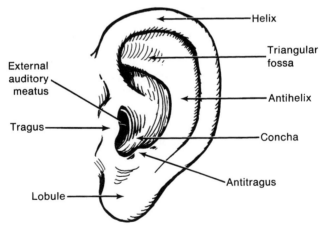

Figure 12-3
Usual landmarks of pinna.
(From Wong DL et al: *Whaley & Wong's nursing care of infants and children,* ed 6, St. Louis, 1999, Mosby.)

Assessment	Findings
	opment and suggests no pathologic process. Skinfolds may be absent from the helix. Parents and child may be sensitive about this abnormality.
Inspect the external ear canal for general hygiene, discharge, and excoriations.	The skin of the external auditory meatus (see Figure 12-3) is normally flesh colored. Soft yellow-brown wax is normal.
	Clinical Alert
	Absence of wax in the external ear may indicate overly vigorous cleaning. Hygienic measures can best be determined by commenting on how clean the ears are and then asking how the ears are cleaned. Parents may need teaching about the dangers of using sharp objects. Advise use of a soft washcloth.
	Absence of wax may also be related to acute otitis media. If cleaning practices are acceptable, ask about ear pulling, irritability, and fever.
	Foul-smelling yellow or green discharge may indicate rupture of a tympanic membrane or recent insertion of myringotomy tubes.
	Bloody discharge may indicate foreign body irritation, scratching, or trauma or rupture of tympanic membrane.
	Serious discharge may indicate allergies.
	Clear discharge may indicate a CSF leak from skull fracture.
Pull on the auricle.	Pulling normally produces no pain and does not produce pain in purulent otitis media.

Assessment	Findings
	Clinical Alert
	Pain produced by pulling on the auricle may indicate otitis externa. Pain will not be produced in purulent otitis media.
Palpate the bony protruberance behind the ear (mastoid) for tenderness.	No pain or tenderness should be experienced when the mastoid is palpated.
	Clinical Alert
	Pain and tenderness over the mastoid process may indicate mastoiditis.

Assessment of Hearing Acuity

Hearing loss, the most common disability, may be of three types. *Conduction hearing loss* results from disruption of sound transmission through the outer and middle ear, most often as the result of serous otitis media. *Sensorineural loss* is a result of damage to the inner ear or auditory nerve. *Mixed loss* reflects both conduction and sensorineural hearing loss.

Assessment	Findings
Infant	
Stand behind the infant and ring a small bell, snap fingers, clap hands, or rustle paper. Be careful not to bump the examining table or to cause an airstream because this evokes a false response from the infant.	The infant younger than 4 months evidences a startle reflex. Infants 6 months of age or older try to locate the sound by shifting their eyes or turning their heads. The infant may also cease sucking or other movement in response to sound.
Assume that parents' impressions of their infant's hearing difficulties are correct unless otherwise proven.	**Clinical Alert**
	Suspect hearing loss in a young infant who does not startle or cease movement or who has been premature and in intensive care.

Assessment	Findings
	Suspect hearing loss in an older infant who does not attempt to localize sound.
	Assume that parents' impressions of their infant's hearing difficulties are correct until otherwise proven.

Preschool-Aged Child

Stand 0.6 to 0.9 m (2 to 3 ft) in front of the child and give commands, such as "Please give me the doll."

School-Aged Child or Adolescent

Stand about 0.3 m (1 ft) behind the child. Instruct the child to cover one ear. Ask the child to repeat what is heard while you whisper numbers in random order. Repeat the process with the other ear.

Rinne's Test
(to compare air and bone conduction)

Strike the tuning fork against your palm, then hold the stem to the child's mastoid process. When the child indicates that the sound is no longer audible, hold the prongs near the external meatus of one ear and ask the child if the sound can be heard. Repeat the process with the other ear.

Not useful in toddlers because the test requires the cooperation and ability of the child to signal when the sound is no longer audible.

Normally the child can hear the sound of the tuning fork at the external meatus after it is no longer audible at the mastoid process (positive test result) because air conduction is better than bone conduction.

Sound should be heard equally well in both ears (positive test result).

Clinical Alert

Interference with conduction of air through the external and middle chambers causes the child to experience sound better through bone conduction.

Assessment	Findings
Weber's Test (to differentiate conduction from sensorineural deafness)	
Strike the tuning fork against the palm and hold the stem in the midline of the child's head. Ask the child where sound is heard best.	**Clinical Alert** With air conduction loss the sound is heard better in the *affected* ear. The sound is heard best in the *unaffected* ear if loss is sensorineural.
Not useful for young children because of difficulty discriminating among "better, more, less."	

Otoscopic Examination

The apprehension many children feel about the otoscopic examination can be lessened by letting them see and handle the otoscope and to turn the light on and off. Reassure that the examination may tickle but does not hurt. Playing a game such as "let's look for the elephant in your ear" may help allay fear (after the examination, it is important to explain that "the elephant" was only pretend). Restrain infants to prevent sudden movement.

Assessment	Findings
Select the largest speculum that fits comfortably into the ear canal. Hold the otoscope in an inverted position.	The ear canal is normally pink, but may be more pigmented in dark-skinned children, and has minute hairs.
Check the canal opening for foreign bodies and scratches.	The tympanic membrane is translucent and pearly pink or gray. Slight redness is normal in newborns and may be normal in older children and infants who have been crying. The tenseness of the membrane causes the otoscopic light to reflect at the 5 o'clock (right ear) or 7 o'clock (left ear) position. The light reflex is a cone-shaped reflection pointing away from the face. The umbo (tip of the malleus) appears as a small, round,
Straighten the ear canal. In children younger than 3 years, pull the earlobe gently down and out. In children older than 3 years, pull the pinna up and back. Place the speculum in the canal. In children younger than 3 years, direct the speculum upward, and in children older than 3 years, direct it downward and forward. Avoid sudden movement. In otoscopes with a	

Assessment	Findings

pneumonic attachment, air can be introduced and removed from the ear canal by squeezing a rubber bulb during otoscopic examination.

Inspect the ear canal for lesions, discharge, cerumen, and foreign bodies.

Inspect the tympanic membrane for bony landmarks, color, fluid level, bubbles, scarring, holes, and vesicles.

concave spot near the middle of the eardrum. The manubrium (handle of the malleus) appears as a whitish line up from the umbo to the membrane margin. A sharp, knob-like protrusion at 1 o'clock represents the short process of the malleus (Figure 12-4).

Clinical Alert

A red, bulging tympanic membrane, dull/absent light reflex, and obscured bony landmarks may indicate acute otitis media (erythema itself does not indicate acute otitis media).

A dull yellow or gray tympanic membrane may indicate serous otitis media.

An ashen gray membrane may suggest scarring from a previous rupture or perforation.

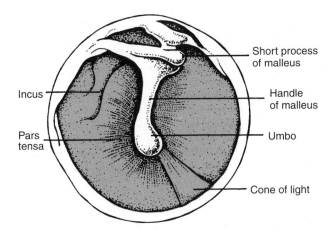

Figure 12-4
Usual landmarks of tympanic membrane.
(From Potter PA: *Pocket guide to health assessment*, ed 4, St. Louis, 1998, Mosby.)

Assessment	Findings
	A black area on the tympanic membrane suggests a perforation that has not yet healed. An area of thin-appearing membrane suggests a healed perforation.
	Absence of movement of the tympanic membrane with the introduction of air may indicate chronic ear infection.
	An apparent line that changes position with movement suggests fluid is present. Circles or rings behind the membrane suggest bubbles in the fluid. Vesicles on the membrane are suggestive of viral infections.

Related Nursing Diagnoses

Impaired comfort: Pain related to infection; pruritus.

Impaired verbal communication: Related to decreased or absent auditory discrimination; decreased or absent auditory comprehension.

Compromised family coping: Related to inability to communicate effectively with child.

Ineffective coping: Related to inability to communicate.

Risk for infection: Secondary to contact with contagious agents.

Risk for injury: Related to knowledge deficit; introduction of foreign objects into ear canal.

Deficient knowledge: Related to appropriate care of the ear.

Impaired parenting: Related to child's inability to communicate; child's inability to hear.

Chronic low self-esteem, disturbance in self-esteem: Related to perception of physical disability.

Disturbed sensory perception: Related to alterations in detection of sound.

Impaired skin integrity: Related to improper cleaning of ear; presence of irritating drainage.

Impaired social interaction: Related to communication difficulties.

Social isolation: Related to hearing loss.

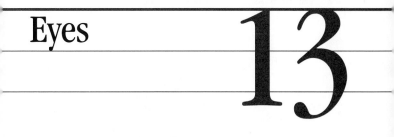

Eyes

Assessment of the eye involves examination of the external and internal eye, visual acuity, extraocular movement, position, alignment, and color vision.

Rationale

Disorders of vision can interfere with a child's ability to respond to stimuli, to learn, and to perform activities of daily living independently. Early detection and referral can minimize the effects of deficiencies in vision. Vision disturbances can alert health practitioners to underlying congenital and acquired disorders.

Anatomy and Physiology

The eye is composed of three layers. The first, outermost layer consists of the sclera, or white of the eye, which is opaque, and of the cornea, which is transparent (Figure 13-1). Underlying the cornea is the iris, which is colored and muscular. At its center is the pupil. The lens lies posterior to the pupil, which is suspended by ciliary muscles. A final layer, the retina, contains rods and cones, which receive visual stimuli and send them to the brain via the optic nerve. The fovea centralis, which appears as a small depression at the back of the retina, contains the most cones. The macula immediately surrounds the fovea centralis. The optic nerve enters the orb through the optic disk. Six muscles hold the eyes in position in their sockets. Coordinated movement of the muscles produces binocular vision. The eyelid, which protects the eye, is lined with the conjunctiva, which is vascular.

At 22 days of gestation the eye appears, and by 8 weeks assumes its familiar form. Its structure and form continue to evolve until the child reaches school age. At birth, myelinization

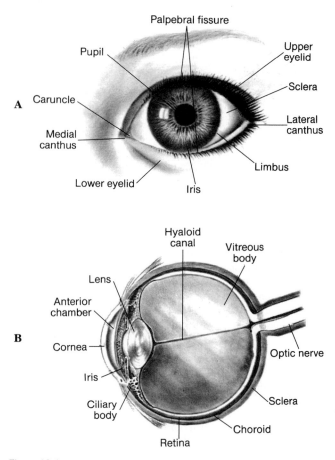

Figure 13-1

Normal structure of eye. **A,** Anterior view. **B,** Cross-sectional view.

(From Wong DL: *Whaley & Wong's nursing care of infants and children,* ed 5, St. Louis, 1995, Mosby.)

of the nerve fibers is complete and a pupillary response can be elicited. The newborn infant, however, has limited vision.

The neonate is able to identify the mother's form and is aware of light and motion, as evidenced by the blink reflex. Searching nystagmus is common. The definitive ability to follow objects is

Table 13-1   Visual Acuity in Infants and Children

Age	Visual Acuity
Birth	Infant fixates on objects 0.2 to 0.3 m (8 to 12 in) away (such as mother's face)
4 mo	20/300 to 20/50
3 yr	±20/40
5 yr	20/30 to 20/20

not developed until about 4 weeks of life, when the infant is able to follow light and objects to midline. By 8 weeks the infant is able to follow light past midline, although strabismus may be evident.

Intermittent convergent strabismus is common until 6 months of age, then disappears. The muscles assume completely mature function by 1 year. The macula and fovea centralis are structurally differentiated by 4 months. Macular maturation is achieved by 6 years of age. Color discrimination is present between 3 and 5 months. The infant is normally farsighted. Like small children, infants see well at close range. Visual acuity in infants ranges from 20/300 to 20/50 (Table 13-1). The iris usually assumes permanent color by 6 months, but in some children not until 1 year. Lacrimation is present by 6 to 12 weeks of age.

Equipment for Eye Assessment

Penlight
Visual acuity chart (choice of chart based on age of child)
    Snellen Letter chart
    Snellen E chart
    Allen cards
Index card
Ophthalmoscope
Ishihara's test (for color vision)
Occluder
Pirate eye patches

Preparation

Ask the parent or child if the child is clumsy, holds books close to eyes, rubs eyes excessively, sits close to the television, has difficulty seeing the board (school-aged child), or responds to approaching objects without blinking (infant). Inquire about school performance; the presence of pain, headache, dizziness, nausea while doing close work; discharge; excessive tearing; squinting; blurred or double vision; burning; itching; and light sensitivity. Inquire whether there is a family history of vision problems (glaucoma, color blindness) and whether the child wears glasses, contact lenses, or a prosthesis. Alert the physician to any of these symptoms.

Assessment of External Eye

Assessment	Findings
Position and Placement	
Note whether the eyes are wide set (hypertelorism) or close set (hypotelorism). Measure the distance between the inner canthi, if in doubt (Figure 13-2).	Inner canthal distance averages 2.5 cm (1 in). **Clinical Alert** Hypertelorism is present in Down syndrome.
Observe for vertical folds that partially or completely cover the inner canthi.	Epicanthal folds are normally seen in Asian children and in some non-Asian children.

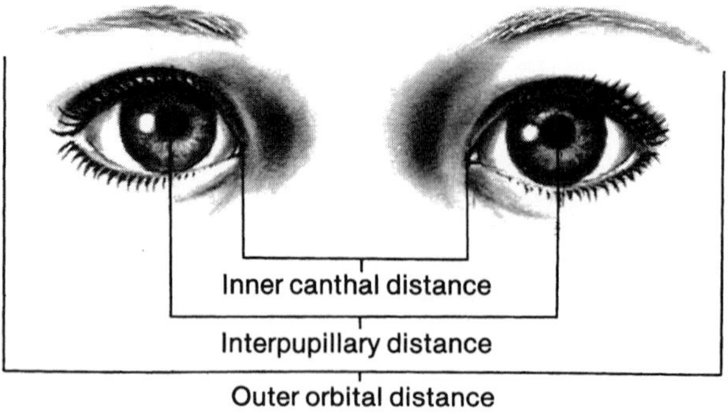

Figure 13-2
Anatomic landmarks of eye.
(From Wong DL et al: *Whaley & Wong's nursing care of infants and children,* ed 6, St. Louis, 1999, Mosby.)

Assessment	Findings
	Clinical Alert
	Epicanthal folds may indicate Down syndrome, renal agenesis, glycogen storage disease, or fetal alcohol syndrome.
Observe the slant of the eyes by drawing an imaginary line across the inner canthi (Figure 13-3).	The palpebral fissures lie horizontally along the imaginary line.
	Asian children normally have an upward slant to their eyes.
	Clinical Alert
	Upward slant of the eyes is present in Down syndrome and may be associated with infants exposed to AIDS/HIV.
	Short palpebral fissures may indicate fetal alcohol syndrome.
Observe the eyelids for proper placement.	The eyelid falls between the upper border of the iris and the upper border of the pupil.
	Clinical Alert
	Appearance of sclera between the upper lid and iris (sunset sign) is present in hydrocephalus, although it may be a normal variant.

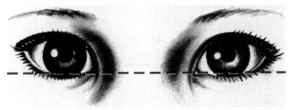

Figure 13-3
Upward palpebral slant.
(From Wong DL et al: *Whaley & Wong's nursing care of infants and children,* ed 6, St. Louis, 1999, Mosby.)

Assessment	Findings
	Drooping of the eyelid over the pupil (ptosis) may be a normal variant or may signal a variety of disorders, such as paralysis of the oculomotor cranial nerve.
	If the eyelids turn inward (entropion), the corners can become irritated by the eyelashes.
	If the eyelids turn outward (ectropion), the conjunctiva is exposed.
	Lid lag and incomplete closure of the eyelid may indicate hyperthyroidism.
Eyebrows	
Inspect the eyebrows for symmetry and hair growth.	Eyebrows normally are shaped and move symmetrically. They do not meet in midline.
Eyelids	
Observe distribution and condition of eyelashes.	Eyelashes curl outward.
Inspect eyelids for color, swelling, discharge, and lesions.	Eyelids normally are the same color as the surrounding skin.
	Clinical Alert
	Flat pink areas on eyelids may be telangiectatic nevi or "stork bite marks," which disappear by 1 year of age.
	A painful, red, swollen eyelid may indicate a stye.
	A nodular nontender area may be a chalazion (cyst).
	Puffiness may be related to thyroid or renal disorders.
	Swelling, redness, and purulent discharge may be related to inflammation of the lacrimal sac (dacryocystitis), often the

Assessment	Findings
	result of a blocked tear duct, which may disappear as an infant reaches 6 months of age.
	If the area around the eyelids appears sunken, the child may be dehydrated.
	Shadow under the eyes may indicate fatigue or allergy.

Conjunctivae

Assessment	Findings
Inspect the lower lid by pulling down as the child looks up. Inspect the upper lid by holding the upper lashes and pulling down and forward gently as the child looks up.	The conjunctivae should be pink and glossy. Yellow striations along the edge are sebaceous glands near the hair follicle. The lacrimal punctum appears as a tiny opening in the medical canthus.
	Clinical Alert
	Redness of the conjunctivae may be related to bacterial or viral infection, allergy, or irritation.
	A cobblestone appearance of the conjunctivae may accompany severe allergy.
	Excessive pallor of the conjunctivae may accompany anemia.
Inspect the bulbar conjunctivae for color.	The bulbar conjunctivae should be clear and transparent, allowing the white of the sclerae to be clearly visible.
	Clinical Alert
	Redness may indicate fatigue, eyestrain, irritation, or bleeding disorders.
	Overgrowth of conjunctival tissue (pterygium) can cover the cornea.
Inspect the sclerae for color.	The sclerae should be white and clear. Tiny black marks in dark-skinned children are normal.

Assessment	Findings
	Clinical Alert Yellow appearance may indicate jaundice. Bluish discoloration may indicate osteogenesis imperfecta, glaucoma, later stages of increased bilirubin, or prenatal exposure to AIDS/HIV.

Pupils and Irises

Assessment	Findings
Inspect the irises for color, shape, and inflammation.	Irises of different colors may be normal. Irises should be round and clear. The cornea covering the iris and pupil should be clear. **Clinical Alert** A notch at the outer edge of the iris (coloboma) may indicate a visual field defect and should be reported. White or light speckling of the iris (Brushfield's spots) may indicate Down syndrome. Absence of color and a pinkish glow may indicate albinism.
Inspect the pupils for size, equality, and response to light. Observe and record the pupil size in normal room light. Darken the room and observe the response of each pupil when light is directly shone into it (direct light reflex) and when light is shone into the opposite eye (consensual light reflex). Place your nondominant hand down the midline of the nose while performing the test for consensual reaction. In infants younger than 5 months, check pupillary reaction by covering	Pupils are normally round and equal in size, although inequality is not uncommon and may be nonpathologic if other findings are normal. Pupils should respond briskly to light. In the consensual reaction the pupil should constrict when light is shone in the contralateral eye. In infants younger than 5 months, pupil inequality is common but should be considered significant if it persists and is accompanied by other central nervous system findings.

Assessment	Findings
each eye with a hand and then uncovering the eye. Pupils that are equal, round, and react to light and accommodation are recorded as PERRLA.	**Clinical Alert** Constriction of the pupils (miosis) may occur with iritis and with morphine administration. Dilation of pupils (mydriasis) may be related to emotional factors, acute glaucoma, some drugs, trauma, circulatory arrest, and anesthesia. Fixed unilateral dilation of a pupil may indicate local eye trauma or head injury.

Assessment of Extraocular Movement

Two tests are commonly used to test binocular vision: the corneal light reflex test and the cover test. The eyes are also assessed for nystagmus (rapid, jerky movements of the eye) through field of vision testing.

Assessment	Findings
Corneal Light Reflex Test	
Assess for strabismus by shining a light directly into the eyes from a distance of about 40.5 cm (16 in). Observe the site of the reflection in each pupil.	Normally the light falls symmetrically on each pupil. Epicanthal folds, often found in Asian children, may give an impression of malalignment. Intermittent alternating convergent strabismus is normal during the first 6 months of life. **Clinical Alert** Report any malalignment. If malalignment is present, the light falls off center in one eye and neither eye deviates. Infants with a birth weight of less than 1500 gm (3.3 lb) are more prone to muscle imbalance and warrant early, periodic screening.

Assessment	Findings

Cover Test

Ask the child to look at your nose; then cover one of the child's eyes. Observe whether the uncovered eye moves. Uncover the occluded eye and inspect for movement.

Clinical Alert
Movement may indicate strabismus. Record the direction of any eye movement. Refer for further testing.

Field of Vision

Ask the child to follow a finger or shiny object through the six cardinal fields of gaze (Figure 13-4). Children younger than 2 or 3 years of age may not be able to cooperate with this test. Observe the eye movements of the younger child as the examination progresses.

A few beats of nystagmus in the far lateral gaze are normal.
Clinical Alert
Report easily elicited nystagmus.

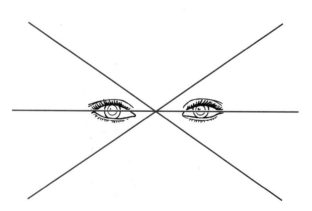

Figure 13-4
Six cardinal fields of gaze.

Assessment of Color Vision

Color vision can be assessed by using Ishihara's test, composed of a set of cards with a series of round dots in the shape of a figure or number. The figures or numbers are not discernible by eyes with impaired color vision.

Assessment of Visual Acuity

Testing of visual acuity in children is not simple and can be directly affected by the child, the nurse, and the environment. There is no simple method to accurately test visual acuity in children younger than 3 years.

Assessment	Findings
Observe whether the infant blinks and exhibits dorsiflexion in response to light.	**Clinical Alert** Report absence of blink reflex.
Observe whether the infant of 4 weeks or older is able to fixate on a brightly colored object and follow it.	**Clinical Alert** Report inability to follow an object and reassess when older.

Snellen's Test

Hang the Snellen chart so that it lies smoothly and firmly on a light-colored wall. There should be no glare on the chart. Have the child stand 6.1 m (20 ft) from the chart. Test both eyes first, then the right eye, then the left eye by having the child cover each eye with an occluder, or with young children, a pirate patch. Unless the child has very poor vision, begin with the line on the chart that corresponds to a distance of 12.2 m (40 ft). The child must be able to see three of four or four of six symbols on a line	**Clinical Alert** Refer children with a two-line difference between eyes, 3-year-old children with a visual acuity of 20/50 or less in either eye, and all other children with 20/40 or less in either eye or who show signs of possible visual disturbances.

Assessment	Findings

to correctly visualize the line. Test with glasses or contact lenses if the child wears them.

If using the Snellen E chart, have the child indicate the direction of the E's "legs" with his/her fingers or with a cardboard E. Use the 20/100 E to determine whether the child understands what to do. Proceed as for regular Snellen testing.

Blackbird Preschool Vision Screening System

Using either the wall-mounted chart or flashcards, ask the child to indicate direction of the bird's flight. This system is useful for nonreaders and children whose first language is not English.

Allen Cards

Show the child the cards at close range and have the child name the pictures from a distance of 4.6 m (15 ft). Test each eye, if possible.

The child should be able to name three of seven cards in a maximum of five tries.

Visual Acuity in Young Infants

Assess for visual acuity in young infants by shining a light into the eyes and noting blinking, pupil constriction, and following of light to midline.

Clinical Alert

Fixed pupils, constant nystagmus, and slow lateral movements may indicate visual loss in young infants.

Ophthalmoscopic Examination

Ophthalmoscopic examination requires practice and patience and a cooperative child. In younger infants and children it may be possible to elicit only the red reflex. The retina, choroid, optic nerve disk, macula, fovea centralis, and retinal vessels are visualized with the ophthalmoscope.

Darken the room. Sit the child on the parent's lap or examination table or lie the child on the table. Use your right hand and eye to examine the child's right eye and your left hand and eye for the left eye. Ask the child to gaze straight ahead.

Assessment	Findings
Set the dial of the ophthalmo-scope at +8 to +2. Approach from a distance of 30.5 cm (12 in), centering the light in the eye. The pupil glows red (red reflex). Gradually move closer and change the dial of the ophthalmoscope to plus or minus diopters to focus.	In infants the optic disk is pale and the peripheral vessels are not well developed. The red reflex appears lighter in infants.
	In children the red reflex appears as a brilliant, uniform glow. The optic disk is creamy white to pinkish, with clear margins. At the center of the optic disk is a small depression (the physiologic cup). Arteries are smaller and brighter than veins. The macula is the same size as the optic disk and located to the right of the disk. The fovea is a glistening spot in the center of the macula.
	Clinical Alert
	Report a partial or white reflex, blurring of the disk margins, bulging of the disk, and hemorrhage.
	Blockage of the red reflex may indicate cataract.
	Papilledema in an older child may indicate acute head injury. Retinal hemorrhage is also associated with acute head injury.

Related Nursing Diagnoses

Impaired comfort: Related to infection; irritation; trauma; strain.

Ineffective coping: Related to temporary or permanent loss of vision.

Deficient diversional activity: Related to inability to perform usual activities of daily living.

Interrupted family processes: Related to disabilities caused by loss of vision.

Delayed growth and development: Related to decreased stimulation secondary to loss of vision.

Risk for infection: Related to contact with contagious elements; loss of integrity of eye tissue.

Risk for injury: Related to inability to see environmental hazards.

Self-care deficit: Related to inability to procure materials needed for self-care; inability to control environment.

Chronic self-esteem: Related to loss of vision; inability to perform self-care.

Disturbed sensory perception: Secondary to trauma; infection; congenital or acquired disorders of vision.

Social isolation: Related to disturbance in self-esteem; inability to control environment; altered interaction.

Face, Nose, and Oral Cavity

14

Rationale

The face provides a map of the child's emotional status and clues to neurologic, congenital, and allergic conditions. The nose provides entry to the respiratory tract, and the mouth provides entry to the digestive tract. Examination of the nose, mouth, and sinuses provides information about the functioning of the respiratory and digestive tracts and about the overall health of the child.

The common occurrence of tonsillitis provides reason enough for inspection of the oropharynx; however, examination of the nose, oral cavity, and oropharynx also yields valuable information about congenital anomalies, nutritional status, hygienic practices, and overall health. The information obtained can be used in the prevention, early detection, and nursing management of such disorders.

Anatomy and Physiology

The face of the newborn infant and child is noticeably different from that of the adult. Typically the neonate appears to have a slightly receding chin. By 6 years of age the mandible and maxilla have grown significantly in length and width and the chin shows greater development. A 6-year-old child has approximately 80% of the facial dimensions of the adult.

Sinuses are air pockets adjacent to the nasal passage. Only the ethmoid and maxillary sinuses are present at birth (Figure 14-1). The frontal sinus develops at around 7 years of age, and the sphenoid sinus develops in adolescence. Development of the sinuses is assisted by enlarging skull bones.

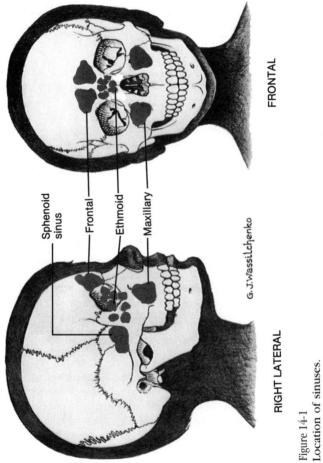

FRONTAL

RIGHT LATERAL

Sphenoid sinus

Frontal

Ethmoid

Maxillary

G.J.Wassilchenko

Figure 14-1
Location of sinuses.
(From Wong DL et al: *Whaley & Wong's nursing care of infants and children,* ed 6, St. Louis, 1999, Mosby.)

The nose warms, filters, and moistens air entering the respiratory tract and is the organ of smell. Infants have a narrow bridge and are obligate nose breathers, which readily predisposes them to compromise of the upper airway. The sense of smell is poor at birth but develops with age.

The mouth of the young infant is short, smooth, and has a relatively long soft palate. The tongue appears large in the shorter oral cavity and tends to press into the concavity of the roof of the mouth, which allows milk to flow back to the pharynx. By 6 months the mouth is proportioned like that of the adult. Until approximately 4 months of age the infant demonstrates an active tongue thrust, or extrusion reflex, in which the tongue is pressed under the nipple. This reflex is of concern to some parents, who think that the infant is rejecting solid foods by thrusting them out as soon as they are placed on the tongue. By approximately 6 months of age the rhythmic up-and-down sucking motions of the tongue become the more adult forward-backward tongue movement. The rooting reflex, in which the infant turns the mouth in the direction that the cheek is touched, assists in food attainment and is seen in the infant younger than 3 or 4 months.

Typically the infant of 3 months begins to drool as salivation increases. The increased saliva production, together with an inappropriate swallowing reflex and lack of lower teeth, allows saliva to flow outward.

The sense of taste is immature at birth but becomes acute by 2 to 3 months as taste buds mature; however, the sense of taste is not fully functional until approximately 2 years of age, as evidenced by the strange things that young children ingest.

In newborn infants the gingivae (gums) are smooth, with a raised fringe of tissue along the gum line. Pear-like areas may be seen along the gingivae. These are often mistaken for teeth, but are retention cysts and disappear in 1 to 2 months. True dentition begins at approximately 6 months of age, when the lower central incisors appear. By 30 months the child has 20 teeth and primary dentition is complete (Figure 14-2). During middle childhood the permanent molars erupt and the primary teeth are lost. The typical 6-year-old appears toothless. Tooth eruptions and losses are genetically predetermined.

Tonsils are found in the pharyngeal cavity and are part of the lymphatic system. Several pairs make up Waldeyer's tonsillar ring, which encircles the pharynx; but only the palatine, or faucial, tonsil

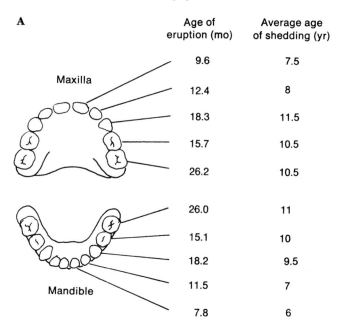

A

	Age of eruption (mo)	Average age of shedding (yr)
Maxilla	9.6	7.5
	12.4	8
	18.3	11.5
	15.7	10.5
	26.2	10.5
	26.0	11
	15.1	10
	18.2	9.5
Mandible	11.5	7
	7.8	6

Figure 14-2
Primary and secondary dentition. **A,** Sequence of eruption and shedding of teeth.
(From Wong DL: *Whaley & Wong's essentials of pediatric nursing,* ed 4, St. Louis, 1993, Mosby.)

is readily visible behind the faucial pillars in the oropharynx (Figure 14-3). The pharyngeal tonsils and adenoids are located on the posterior wall of the oropharynx. Although tonsillar tissue begins to shrink by approximately 7 years of age, the child normally has larger tonsils and adenoids than either the infant or the adolescent.

Equipment for Face, Nose, and Oral Cavity Assessment

Tongue blade (flavored, if available)
Penlight
Glove

B

Average age
of eruption (yr)

Central incisor	7.35
Lateral incisor	8.45
Cuspid	11.35
First bicuspid	10.2
Second bicuspid	11.05
First molar	6.3
Second molar	12.25
Third molar	Variable 17-21
Third molar	
Second molar	11.9
First molar	6.05
Second bicuspid	11.2
First bicuspid	10.5
Cuspid	10.35
Lateral incisor	7.5
Central incisor	6.4

Maxilla

Mandible

Figure 14-2, cont'd
B, Sequence of eruption of secondary teeth.

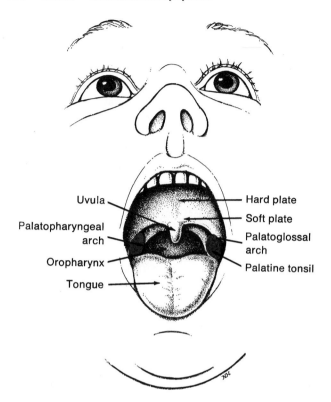

Figure 14-3
Interior structures of mouth.
(From Wong DL et al: *Whaley & Wong's nursing care of infants and children,*
ed 6, St. Louis, 1999, Mosby.)

Preparation

Inquire whether the child has or has had frequent sore throats,
epistaxis, allergies, hay fever, recent contacts with persons with
communicable disease, fever, difficulty in swallowing, or vocal
changes (e.g., hoarseness or nasality). Ask about oral hygiene
practices and date of last dental visit (if 3 years or older). Ask if the
child is receiving medications.

   Infants and children find examination of the mouth intrusive,
and it is best left until the end of the examination. The nurse often

has an opportunity to visualize the oral cavity without a tongue blade when the infant or child cries, laughs, or yawns. Infants and young children are often more comfortable on the parent's lap during this part of the examination and can be reclined slightly for a better view. Infants and young children may need restraining.

Assessment of Face and Nose

Assessment	Findings
Observe the spacing and size of facial features.	Infants who were premature may have a narrow forehead. **Clinical Alert** Coarse features combined with a low hairline and large tongue may indicate cretinism. An enlarged forehead may indicate hydrocephalus or ectodermal dysplasia.
Carefully observe the facial expression, especially around the eyes and mouth.	**Clinical Alert** A child with a persistently sad and forlorn expression may be abused, particularly if bruises can be detected on the body. A child who demonstrates an open mouth and facial contortions may be suffering from allergic rhinitis. Shadows under the eyes may indicate fatigue or allergy.
Observe the symmetry of the nasolabial folds as the child cries and smiles.	Normal nasolabial folds are symmetric. **Clinical Alert** Asymmetry of the nasolabial folds may indicate facial nerve impairment or Bell's palsy.
Tilt the head backward and push the tip of the nose upward to visualize the internal nasal cavity. Use a penlight for better illumination. Observe the	The nasal mucosa should be firm and pink. **Clinical Alert** A pale, boggy nasal mucosa, with or without pink-grape

Assessment	Findings
integrity, color, and consistency of the mucosa, the position of the septum, and for perforation of the septum. Perforation will be indicated by light showing through the perforation to the other nostril.	polyps, indicates allergic rhinitis. A red mucosa indicates infection. Excoriation of the nasal mucosa may indicate nose picking, a common cause of epistaxis in children, or cocaine use. Grayish soft outgrowths of mucosa are polyps that may partially obstruct the nares. Report any deviation of the nasal septum. Diminished nasal hair may suggest cocaine use.
Ask older children about their sense of smell. Test the sense of smell by having the child close his or her eyes. Block one nostril at a time and ask the child to identify distinctive odors such as coffee and lemon. The child should be able to correctly identify each.	**Clinical Alert** Diminished smell may indicate olfactory nerve impairment.
Palpate above the eyebrows and each side of the nose to determine if pain and tenderness are present.	**Clinical Alert** Pain and tenderness in these regions may indicate sinusitis.

Related Nursing Diagnoses

Ineffective airway clearance: Related to decreased nasal patency; swollen mucous membranes.

Anxiety: Related to air hunger.

Risk for infection: Related to contact with contagious agents.

Disturbed sensory perception: Secondary to olfactory nerve impairment; obstruction; sinusitis.

Impaired skin integrity: Related to irritating nasal secretions.

Assessment of Oral Cavity

Assessment	Findings
Inspect the lips for color, symmetry, moisture, swelling, sores, and fissures.	The lips should be intact, pink, and firm. **Clinical Alert** Blueness of the lips is a reliable sign of cyanosis in white children. Deep red coloration may be present in an asthmatic attack. Pallor may indicate anemia. Cherry red coloration is seen with acidosis. Cracked lips are usually the result of harsh climate, lip biting, mouth breathing, or fever. Fissures at the corners of the mouth may indicate deficiency of riboflavin or niacin. Drooping of one side of the lips indicates facial nerve impairment. A thin upper lip and long philtrum may suggest fetal alcohol syndrome, if other features of the syndrome are present.
Inspect the buccal margins, gingivae, tongue, and palate for moisture, color, intactness, and bleeding. To inspect the buccal mucosa, ask the child to use his or her fingers to move the outer lip and cheek to one side. With toddlers and infants, it is necessary to use a tongue blade, unless a good view is possible while the child is crying. When using the tongue blade, slide it along the side of the tongue.	The oral membranes are normally pink, firm, smooth, and moist. The buccal cavity, tongue margins, and gums appear bluish in black children.

Assessment	Findings
Use a glove and penlight for clearer visualization of any suspected abnormalities.	**Clinical Alert**
Observe for the presence of odor or halitosis.	White ulcerated sores on the oral mucosa are cankers, related to mild trauma, viral infection, or local irritants.

Clinical Alert

White ulcerated sores on the oral mucosa are cankers, related to mild trauma, viral infection, or local irritants.

Salt-like areas rimmed with red and found on the inner cheek opposite the second molar are Koplik's spots and indicate the onset of measles.

White curdy patches on the gum margins, inner cheeks, tongue, or palate usually indicate thrush (oral monilia-sis). Thrush is common in infants (particularly during or following antibiotic therapy), but in children could indicate a deficient immune system disorder such as AIDS or infection with HIV. These patches may be distinguished from milk curds in that they cannot be easily scraped away.

Hyperplasic gum tissue may be related to anticonvulsant therapy.

Reddened, swollen, bleeding gums may indicate infection, poor nutrition, or poor oral hygiene.

A red tongue is related to vitamin deficiencies and to scarlet fever ("strawberry tongue").

Dry, sticky mucous membranes suggest dehydration.

Assessment	Findings
Observe the size and shape of the nose. Draw an imaginary line down the center of the face between the eyes and down the notch of the upper lip.	The nose should be symmetric and in the center of the face. A flattened bridge is sometimes seen in Asian and black children. **Clinical Alert** A flattened nose may indicate congenital anomalies and should be reported.
Observe the external nares for flaring, discharge, excoriation, and odor.	**Clinical Alert** Flaring external nares indicate respiratory distress. The skin of the external nares should be intact. No discharge should be seen, although a clear, watery discharge may be present if the child has been crying. Excoriation of the external nares may indicate the presence of an irritating discharge and frequent nose wiping. A clear, thin, nasal discharge is often present with allergic rhinitis. Purulent yellow or green discharge accompanies infection. Clear nasal discharge that tests positive for glucose (as tested with Dextrostix) following a head injury may suggest leakage of spinal fluid from a skull fracture. A foul odor may indicate the presence of a foreign body.
Test the patency of the nares by placing the diaphragm of the stethoscope under one nostril while blocking the other. A film appears on the diaphragm if the naris is patent.	Both nares should be patent. **Clinical Alert** A gray, furrowed tongue may be normal or may indicate drug ingestion, allergy, or fever.

Assessment	Findings
	Clefts or notches in the hard or soft palate should be noted. An abnormally high, narrow arch may cause problems with sucking in the infant and with speech in the older child.
	Petechiae on oral mucous membranes may indicate presence of emboli, accidental biting, or infection.
	Odor or halitosis can indicate poor oral hygiene, constipation, dehydration, sinusitis, food trapped in tonsillar crypts, or systemic illness.
	Drooling accompanied by fever and respiratory distress is indicative of epiglottitis.
Inspect the tongue for movement and size. The older child can be asked to reach the tip of the tongue to the roof of the mouth.	The frenulum attaches to the undersurface of the tongue or near its tip, allowing the child to reach the areolar ridge with the tip of the tongue.
Observe the movement of the tongue in infants and younger children as they vocalize or cry.	**Clinical Alert**
	Inability to touch the tongue to the areolar ridge may signify tongue tie and later speech problems.
	Glossoptosis, or tongue protrusion, is seen in mental retardation and cerebral palsy.
Inspect the teeth for number, type, condition, and occlusion. To estimate the number of teeth that should be present in a child 2 years of age or younger, subtract 6 months from the child's age in months. Ask the child who is 5 years or older if	A normal 30-month-old child has 20 temporary teeth. A child with full permanent dentition has 32 teeth. The upper teeth should slightly override the lower teeth.
	Clinical Alert
	Brown and black spots usually indicate caries. Mottling may

Assessment	Findings
teeth are loose. To assess malocclusion, ask the child to bite down hard.	indicate excessive fluoride intake. Green and black staining can accompany oral iron intake.
	Extensive decay of the maxillary or upper incisors and molars in infants and young children suggests nursing or bottle caries.
	An increase in dental caries in adolescents may indicate frequent, self-induced vomiting.
	Absent, delayed, or pegteeth may indicate ectodermal dysplasia.
	Protrusion of the lower teeth or marked protrusion of the upper teeth should be noted.
Tonsils may be inspected in the older child by asking the child to say "ahh" or to yawn. Asking the child to tilt the head slightly back, to breathe deeply, and to hold the breath can also aid in visualization. If the child has difficulty holding the tongue down, the tongue can be *lightly* depressed with the tongue blade on either side. Playing games and demonstrating what is expected of the child through the use of a parent or doll can be very useful. If the nurse is unable to observe the tonsil bed while the infant or older child is crying, the tongue blade can be slid between the lips, along the side of the gum, then quickly slipped between	Tonsils, if present, are normally the same color as the buccal mucosa. They are large in the preschool- and school-aged child and appear larger as they move toward the uvula. Crypts may be present on their surface.
	Clinical Alert
	Reddened tonsils covered with white exudate suggest group A β-hemolytic streptococcal infection or infectious mononucleosis.
	Thick, gray, exudate may indicate diphtheric tonsillitis.
	Visualization of adenoids suggests that they are enlarged. If adenoids are visualized during gagging or saying "ahh," they appear as grapelike structures.

Assessment	Findings
the gums along the side of the tongue. *Any inspection of the pharynx that involves use of the tongue blade and that may elicit the gag reflex must not be performed in a child who is suspected to have any of the croup syndromes.*	
Observe movement of the uvula during examination of the tonsils. Movement of the uvula can be assessed by producing a gag reflex.	The uvula remains in midline. Upon gagging the uvula moves upward. **Clinical Alert** Deviation of the uvula or absence of movement may signal involvement of the glossopharyngeal or vagus nerves. Producing the gag reflex in a child with epiglottitis could produce total obstruction.
Observe the quality of the voice.	**Clinical Alert** A nasal quality to the voice suggests enlarged adenoids. A hoarse cry or voice may indicate croup, cretinism, tetany, or congenital hypothyroidism. A shrill, high-pitched cry may indicate increased intracranial pressure.

Related Nursing Diagnoses

Ineffective airway clearance: Related to swelling.

Impaired comfort: Pain related to infection; inflammation.

Impaired verbal communication: Related to pain; anxiety; tongue tie; inflammation.

Compromised family coping: Related to situational crisis; anxiety.

Impaired dentition: Related to neglect of hygiene; feeding practices; lack of knowledge.

Deficient fluid volume: Related to reluctance to drink; inability to swallow secondary to pain and swelling.

Infection: Related to contact with contagious agents.

Deficient knowledge: Related to oral hygiene; alleviation of symptoms of respiratory distress.

Imbalanced nutrition: Less than body requirements related to increased metabolic needs; reluctance or inability to swallow; loss of tissue integrity.

Impaired oral mucous membranes: Related to infection; fever; dehydration.

Disturbed sensory perception: Related to infection; diminished taste.

Impaired swallowing: Related to pain; swelling; neuromuscular dysfunction.

Thorax
and Lungs

15

Assessment of the respiratory system includes close observation of the child's behavior and assessment of the thorax and the anterior and posterior chest.

Rationale

Respiratory disorders are common in infancy and in childhood and can be acute, life threatening, or chronic. Early screening and detection are essential to being able to refer children for medical treatment. Knowledgeable assessment also assists in monitoring the progress of treatment.

Anatomy and Physiology

Lungs have two main functions: to supply the body with oxygen and eliminate carbon dioxide and to maintain the body's acid-base balance. The lungs are paired and symmetric. The right lung has three lobes, and the left lung has two lobes. Air enters the lungs via the trachea and larynx from the mouth or nose. The trachea branches into two major bronchi. The right bronchus is shorter, wider, and angled less sharply to the side than the left.

Fetal lung buds first arise in the first lunar month of gestation, along with nasal pits, the trachea, and the larynx. Subsequent budding and branching create the mainstem bronchi pulmonary lobules in the second month. Branching continues into early childhood, although it is less proliferative. By the third month, elementary respiratory-like movements are observed. From the sixth month on, the lobules have developed alveolar ducts, and the ducts have developed alveoli.

As the alveolar sacs develop, the epithelium lining the sacs thins. Pulmonary capillaries press into the walls of the sacs as the lungs are prepared for the exchange of oxygen and carbon dioxide, near the end of the sixth month of gestation. During the final weeks of gestation the lungs secrete surfactants that reduce the surface tension of the alveolar sacs and prevent the alveoli from collapsing and producing atelectasis. At birth, the lungs are fluid filled. This fluid is rapidly dispelled and absorbed as the lungs fill with air.

The newborn infant's thoracic cage is nearly round. Gradually the transverse diameter increases until the chest assumes the elliptic shape of the adult, at about 6 years of age. The infant's thoracic cage is also relatively soft, which allows the cage to pull in during labored breathing. Infants have relatively less tissue and cartilage in the trachea and bronchi, which allows these structures to collapse more readily.

Airways tend to grow faster than the vertebral column. In infancy the bifurcation of the trachea is at the level of the third thoracic vertebra. By adulthood the bifurcation is at the level of the fourth thoracic vertebra. Smaller airways in young children and infants tend to narrow more readily from edema and secretions than in older children and adolescents. Shorter distances between structures in the young child also contribute to rapid transmission of organisms and widespread involvement.

Young infants (up to 6 months) are obligatory nose breathers, and their nasal passages are narrower. Breathing is less rhythmic than in the child. In infants and children younger than 6 or 7 years, respirations are chiefly diaphragmatic or abdominal; in older children and especially females, respirations are chiefly thoracic. The volume of oxygen expired by the infant and the child is greater than that expired by the adult. The volume of air that is inspired increases as the child grows. At the age of 12 years the child has approximately nine times the number of alveoli that were present at birth.

As with heart rate, the respiratory rate in infants and children responds more dramatically than in adults to emotion, illness, and exercise. The rate tends to show greater variability and wider range than with adults.

Equipment for Assessment of Thorax and Lungs

Stethoscope
Pulse oximeter

Preparation

Ask the parent or child about cough, fever, shortness of breath, difficulty in breathing, wheezing, easy fatigability, meningeal signs, abdominal pain, vomiting, sore throat, past respiratory tract infections, frequent colds, family history of respiratory disorders and smoking, history of allergies, immunization status, and type of childcare setting (e.g., home, daycare).

Allow the younger child to play with the stethoscope before performing the assessment. Children often enjoy listening to the sounds in their chests and in their parents' or the nurse's chest. Remove the child's shirt or blouse for best visualization of the chest. Infants and toddlers are often best assessed while held by their parents.

Assessment of Thorax and Lungs

Assessment	Findings
Assess for stridor (high-pitched crowing sound), grunting, hoarseness, snoring, audible wheezing, and cough (Table 15-1). Precisely describe the sounds and their occurrence.	**Clinical Alert** Stridor, hoarseness, and a barking cough accompany croup syndromes. Inspiratory stridor and expiratory snoring are indicative of epiglottis. Wheezing may indicate asthma, respiratory syncytial virus, or foreign body aspiration. Short, rapid coughs followed by a crowing sound or whoop is indicative of whooping cough.
Observe the external nares for flaring.	**Clinical Alert** Flaring indicates respiratory distress.
Observe the nailbeds for color and for clubbing (widening and lengthening) of the terminal phalanges (Figure 15-1).	**Clinical Alert** Cyanosis (bluish coloration of nailbeds) is sometimes indicative of respiratory failure. Cyanosis may also be related to vasoconstriction or polycythemia.

Text continued on p. 170

Table 15-1 Characteristics and Common Etiologies of Cough in Infants and Children

Characteristics of Cough	Pattern and Progression of Cough	Fever	Common Age-Group Affected	Associated Symptoms	Possible Etiology
Dry, hacking	May become productive of mucoid or blood-streaked sputum	Low-grade to high	Any	• Headache • Malaise • Dyspnea • Fine rales	Viral pneumonia
Dry, hacking, harsh	More pronounced than with common cold. Tends to become more persistent and annoying by end of second week. May progress to paroxysmal stage, where cough involves explosive bursts on expiration, followed by an inspiratory "whoop." Coughing may be precipitated by eating or drinking, especially milk.	None to low-grade	Any but primarily in children younger than 4 years, who have not been immunized	• Copious lacrimation and coryza • Looks distressed while coughing; face becomes red or cyanotic • Eyes prominent while coughing • May have retinal hemorrhages • Vomits thick, tenacious material with coughing	Pertussis (whooping cough)

Continued

Table 15-1 Characteristics and Common Etiologies of Cough in Infants and Children—cont'd

Characteristics of Cough	Pattern and Progression of Cough	Fever	Common Age Group Affected	Associated Symptoms	Possible Etiology
Dry, irritated	Persistent	Absent	May accompany allergic manifestations or be present in child with family history of allergies	• Clear nasal discharge • Sneezing • Conjunctivitis	Allergic cough
Dry, hacking	Worse at night; productive in 2 to 3 days	Moderate	First 4 years of life; may also be found in teens using marijuana.	• Upper respiratory infection	Bronchitis
Dry, nonproductive	Becomes paroxysmal with mucus production	None, unless infection present	Onset before 3 years	• Chronic rhinitis • Chronic sinusitis • Chronic respiratory infections • Failure to thrive • Clubbing of fingers and toes • Increasing dyspnea and wheezing	Cystic fibrosis

				• Barrel chest • Numerous other symptoms associated with involvement of gastrointestinal and other systems	
Brassy	Slowly progressive	Low grade	3 months to 8 years	• Hoarseness • Dyspnea • Restlessness	Acute laryngotracheobronchitis
Croupy	Sudden onset; common at night	High	3 months to 3 years	• Stridor • Hoarseness • Restlessness • Upper respiratory infection • Recurs	Acute spasmodic laryngitis (spasmodic croup)
Croupy	Moderately progressive with purulent secretions	High	1 month to 6 years	• Stridor • Upper respiratory infection	Acute tracheitis

Continued

Table 15-1 Characteristics and Common Etiologies of Cough in Infants and Children—cont'd

Characteristics of Cough	Pattern and Progression of Cough	Fever	Common Age-Group Affected	Associated Symptoms	Possible Etiology
Paroxysmal, nonproductive	Mild symptoms at first, progressing to paroxysmal cough and sometimes wheezing	High	2 to 12 months	• Rhinorrhea • Pharyngitis • Air hunger • Tachypnea • Cyanosis • Apneic spells	Respiratory syncytial virus
Hacking, wheezing, productive	Cough can produce frothy, clear, gelatinous sputum	Absent	Onset 1 to 5 years	• Audible wheeze • Prolonged expiratory phase • Malar flush and red ears • Chest hyperresonant	Asthma

| Productive cough | Progressive; productive of mucoid, purulent, blood-streaked, or rusty sputum | High | Any | • Older children may sit upright, shoulders forward
• Exhaustion
• Abrupt onset
• Chills
• Headache
• Neck stiffness
• Chest pain exaggerated by deep breathing
• Abdominal discomfort
• Malaise
• Rapid, shallow respirations | Bacterial pneumonia |

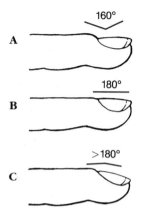

Figure 15-1
Clubbing of nails. **A,** Normal nail. Angle between nail and nail base is approximately 160 degrees. **B,** Early clubbing. Angle between nail and nail base is almost 180 degrees, caused by tissue proliferation on terminal phalanx. **C,** Late clubbing. Angle between nail and nail base is less than 180 degrees. Nail base is visibly swollen.

Assessment	Findings
	Clubbing usually indicates chronic hypoxemia, as in cystic fibrosis and bronchiectasis.
Evaluate oxygen saturation levels through pulse oximetry. If using fingers for sensor placement, remove nail polish because it can distort readings. Placement distal to a blood pressure cuff may also distort readings.	
Observe the color of the child's trunk.	**Clinical Alert** Mottling and cyanosis of the trunk indicate severe hypoxemia.

Assessment	Findings
Inspect the thorax for configuration, symmetry, and abnormalities. Measure the size of the chest by placing a tape around the chest at the nipple line. For greatest accuracy, record measurement during inspiration and expiration and average the two. Chest size is largely important in relation to head circumference in infants.	The chest is rounder in young children. By 6 years of age the ratio of anteroposterior diameter to transverse diameter is about 1:35.
	In some infants the sternum may be so pliant that the chest appears to cave in with each breath.
	The thorax should move symmetrically.
	Clinical Alert
	A round chest in an older child usually indicates a chronic lung disorder.
	A protruberant sternum (pectus carinatum, or pigeon breast) or depressed sternum (pectus excavatum) should be noted. Either may compromise lung expansion.
	Decreased movement of one side of the thorax may indicate pneumonia, pneumothorax, or a foreign body.
	Enlargement of one side of the thorax may indicate a diaphragmatic hernia. Enlargement of the left side may indicate an enlarged heart.
Note the size of the breasts in relation to the age of the child.	Enlarged breasts may be seen in the young infant as a result of maternal hormonal influences.
	Clinical Alert
	Enlarged breasts (gynecomastia) in older male children may indicate obesity or hormonal or systemic problems.

Assessment	Findings
Observe the chest for retractions, or indrawings, in the supraclavicular (above the clavicles), tracheal (in the sternal notch), substernal (below the sternum), and intercostal (between the ribs) areas (Figure 15-2). Puffiness or bulging of these areas may also be present.	**Clinical Alert** Retractions indicate labored breathing in infants and children. Puffiness accompanies severe air trapping. Extension of the head on inspiration may indicate use of accessory muscles and of severe respiratory disease in infants.
Observe the child for type of breathing.	In children younger than 7 years respirations are diaphragmatic, and the abdomen rises with inspiration. In girls older than 7 years breathing becomes

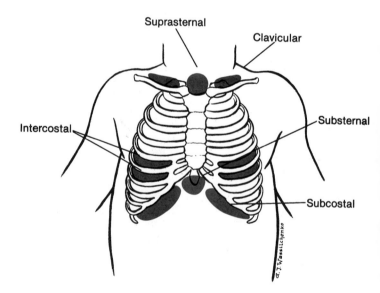

Figure 15-2
Areas where retractions are found.
(From Wong DL et al: *Whaley & Wong's nursing care of infants and children,* ed 6, St. Louis, 1999, Mosby.)

Assessment	Findings
	thoracic. Abdomen and chest should move together regardless of type of breathing.
	Clinical Alert
	Abdominal breathing in an older child may indicate a respiratory disorder or fractured rib. In labored abdominal breathing the abdomen pushes out abruptly.
Observe the depth and regularity of respirations and the duration of inspiration in relation to expiration.	**Clinical Alert**
	A prolonged expiratory phase may indicate an obstructive respiratory problem, such as asthma.

Palpation

To assess respiratory excursion, place your hands, thumbs together, along the costal margins of the child's chest or back while the child is sitting.	Movement is symmetric with each breath. Posterior base descends approximately 6 cm (2.3 in) during deep inspiration.
Palpate for tactile fremitus by using either the fingertips or the palmar surfaces of your hands. Move symmetrically while the child says "99" or "blue moon." In the infant, fremitus may be felt as the infant cries.	Fremitus is normally less at the base of the lung.
	Clinical Alert
	Decreased fremitus may indicate asthma, pneumothorax, or a foreign body.
	Increased fremitus occurs with pneumonia and atelectasis.

Percussion

Percussion is more useful in older children.	Resonance (a low, long sound) it heard over all lung surfaces.
Using the indirect method, percuss the anterior and posterior chest.	Dullness may be heard over the fifth right intercostal space, because of the liver, and over the second to fifth left intercostal space, because of the heart.
Percuss over the intercostal spaces, moving symmetrically and systematically. The child	

Assessment	Findings
may sit or lie while the anterior chest is percussed, and sit while the posterior chest is percussed.	Tympany (a loud, musical sound) may be heard over the sixth left intercostal space. **Clinical Alert** The percussion note is dull if fluid or a mass is present in the lungs. Hyperresonance occurs during an asthmatic episode.

Auscultation

Assessment	Findings
Using the warmed diaphragm and bell of the stethoscope, auscultate the lung fields systematically and *symmetrically* from apex to base. The bell is used for low-pitched sounds, the diaphragm for higher-pitched sounds.	Breath sounds (Table 15-2) normally seem louder and harsher in the infant and young child because of the thinness of the chest wall. **Clinical Alert** Report any adventitious sounds (Table 15-3 on pg. 176) or breath sounds heard in other than expected areas. If unable to name the sound heard, describe it. Asymmetric rhonchi or wheezes may signal presence of a foreign body.
Use a pediatric diaphragm or the bell for infants and small children. Children can be encouraged to breathe deeply by pretending to blow up balloons or blow out candles, or by blowing away a piece of tissue or cotton ball.	
Auscultate the axillae of children with pneumonia. Rales or crackles may be easily heard in these areas.	Unilaterally absent breath sounds may indicate pneumothorax. In infants, breath sounds may be diminished, and not absent, in pneumothorax.
Sounds may be referred from the upper respiratory tract if a child has mucus in the nose or throat. To determine if sounds are referred, place the diaphragm near the child's mouth. Referred sounds are loudest near their origin and are symmetrical.	Inaudible breath sounds and crackles may indicate severe spasm or obstruction during an asthmatic episode.

Table 15-2 Breath Sounds

Sound	Relationship of Inspiration to Expiration	Diagram of Sound	Location Normal	Location Abnormal
Vesicular	Inspiration > Expiration		Throughout lung field	None
Bronchovesicular	Inspiration = Expiration		First or second intercostal space, at level of bifurcation of trachea	Peripheral lung
Bronchotubular	Inspiration < Expiration		Over trachea	Lung area

Table 15-3 Adventitious Sounds

Sound	Characteristics	Cause
Crackles (rales)		
Fine	Intermittent, high-pitched, soft popping sounds. Heard late in inspiration. Indicative of fluid in alveoli. May be normal in newborns and older infants.	Pneumonia, congestive heart failure, tuberculosis
Medium	Intermittent, wet, loud, noncrackling, medium pitched. Heard in early or mid-inspiration. Clear with coughing. Indicative of fluid in bronchioles and bronchi.	Pulmonary edema
Coarse	Loud, bubbling, low pitched. Heard on expiration. Clear with coughing. Indicative of fluid in bronchioles and bronchi.	Resolving pneumonia, bronchitis
Rhonchus	Continuous, snoring, low pitched. Heard throughout respiratory cycle. Clear with coughing. Indicative of involvement of large bronchi and trachea. May also be normal.	Bronchitis
Wheeze	Continuous, musical, high pitched. Heard in middle to late expiration. Indicative of edema and obstruction in smaller airways. May be audible without a stethoscope.	Asthma
Audible wheezes		
Inspiratory	Sonorous, musical. Heard on inspiration.	High obstruction
Expiratory	Whistling, sighing. Heard during expiration.	Low obstruction
Pleural friction rub	Grating, rubbing, loud, high pitched. May be heard during both inspiration and expiration.	Inflamed pleural surfaces
Crepitation	Coarse, cracking sensation as hand passes over affected area.	Injury, surgical intervention

Related Nursing Diagnoses

Activity intolerance: Related to breathlessness; fatigue secondary to respiratory infection or obstruction.

Ineffective airway clearance: Related to secretions; physical alterations of the chest wall; limited expansion of the chest wall.

Anxiety: Related to breathlessness.

Risk for imbalanced body temperature: Related to infection; inflammation.

Fear: Related to loss of control; air hunger.

Impaired gas exchange: Related to exudate; swelling; obstruction.

Delayed growth and development: impaired related to chronic lack of oxygen.

Impaired home maintenance: Related to home oxygen therapy; medication administration.

Risk for infection: Related to contact with contagious agents.

Deficient knowledge: Related to therapies; medication; recognition of symptoms.

Impaired parenting: Related to situational crisis.

Sleep deprivation: Related to air hunger; cough.

Ineffective tissue perfusion: Cardiopulmonary related to swelling and exudate secondary to infection and inflammation.

Cardiovascular System 16

The heart is the primary focus of cardiovascular assessment in the infant and child. Assessment of peripheral circulation may be necessitated under conditions such as application of casts. Auscultation provides the most significant data on cardiac status and receives the most emphasis, yet the importance of other assessments cannot be overlooked.

Rationale

It is estimated that 50% of all children have innocent heart murmurs. Screening and referral of children with murmurs assists in distinguishing between innocent and organic murmurs. Assessment of cardiac and vascular function is an essential component of many hospitalizations, particularly when surgery is performed and when drugs are administered. When cardiac problems have been identified, knowledgeable assessment aids in monitoring the effectiveness of treatment regimens and in early detection of complications.

Anatomy and Physiology

The heart is a muscular four-chambered organ located in the mediastinum. The upper chambers of the heart are the atria, and the lower chambers are the ventricles. Septa divide the two ventricles and the two atria. Four valves prevent the backflow of blood into the chambers. The tricuspid valve, located between the right atrium and ventricle, and the bicuspid, or mitral valve, located between the left atrium and ventricle, are the atrioventricular valves. The pulmonic valve, located in the pulmonary artery, and the aortic valve, in the aorta, are the semilunar valves. Closure of the four valves produces vibrations that are thought to be responsible for heart sounds. S_1 refers to the "lubb" sound produced by closure of the atrioventricular valves, and S_2 to the "dubb" sound produced by closure of the semilunar valves. Table 16-1 summarizes the various sounds and their characteristics.

In its initial stage of development the heart is a straight tube. Between the second and tenth weeks of gestation it undergoes a series of changes to become a four-chambered organ. The heart begins beating during the third week of gestation. During fetal life it primarily distributes the oxygen and nutrients that have been supplied through the placenta. The fetal lungs are largely bypassed by shunts that exist during fetal life. At birth these shunts begin to close as pulmonary vascular resistance drops. Pulmonary vascular resistance approximates adult levels by 6 weeks. Pulmonary vascular resistance is still relatively high in the first month of life, and cardiac defects such as ventricular septal defect may not be detected.

The heart is large in relation to body size in the infant. It lies somewhat horizontally and occupies a larger portion of the thoracic cavity. Growth of the lungs causes the heart to assume a lower position, and by 7 years of age the heart has assumed an adult position that is more oblique and lower. Heart size increases in adolescence in conjunction with rapid growth.

At birth ventricular walls are similar in thickness, but with circulatory demands the left ventricle increases in thickness. The thinness of the ventricle produces a low systolic pressure in the newborn. The systolic pressure rises after birth until it approximates adult levels by puberty. Blood vessels lengthen and thicken in response to increased pressures.

Equipment for Assessment of Cardiovascular System

Stethoscope (preferably with a small diaphragm)

Preparation

The child may sit or lie. Allow the child to handle the stethoscope. Listening to the parent's or nurse's heart or to their own hearts is often effective in dispelling anxieties in young patients. Ask the parent or child about heart disease in family members. Inquire whether the child has had difficulty in feeding (infant), undue fatigue, intolerance for exercise, poor weight gain, weakness,

Table 16-1   **Heart Sounds**

Sound	Cause	Location	Characteristic
S_1 (lubb)	Mitral and tricuspid valves are forced closed at the beginning of systole (contraction).	Apex of heart	S_1 is longer and lower pitched than S_2. Synchronous with carotid pulse. Closure of valves usually heard as one sound, but slight asynchrony may produce audible splitting, best heard in the fourth left interspace.
S_2 (dubb)	Aortic and pulmonic valves are forced closed at the beginning of diastole (heart relaxation).	Base of heart	Short, high-pitched S_2 may be split during inspiration. Splitting is best heard in the aortic area. If the breath is held on inspiration, "physiologic split" is accentuated.
S_3	Vibrations are produced by rapid ventricular filling.	Apex of heart	Heard early in diastole. Dull, low-pitched. Normal in children and young adults.
S_4	Resistance to ventricular filling after contraction of atria.	Apex of heart	Low pitched. Considered abnormal. Best heard when child is supine.

cyanosis, edema, dizziness, epistaxis, squatting, frequent respiratory tract infections, or delayed development. Ask the parent whether the mother had any infection or took medications during pregnancy, age of mother at infant's birth, and presence of maternal diabetes or alcohol use. Inquire whether the child had problems at birth, such as low birth weight, prematurity, congenital infection, or respiratory difficulty. Inquire about temperament of the child and family responses to illness.

Assessment of Heart

Assessment	Findings
Inspection	
Observe the child's body posture.	**Clinical Alert**
	Squatting is seen in tetralogy of Fallot.
	Persistent slight hyperextension of the neck in infants may indicate hypoxia.
	Restlessness accompanied by abdominal pain, pallor, vomiting, unconsolable crying, and shock may indicate acute myocardial infarction in susceptible children.
Observe the child for cyanosis, mottling, and edema.	**Clinical Alert**
	Cyanosis, pallor, and mottling may indicate heart disease. Edema may indicate congestive heart failure. Edema of sacral and periorbital areas is more common in younger children. Edema of the extremities is more common in older children, but in the younger child may more likely indicate renal failure.
	Cyanosis increases with crying in children with an atrioventricular canal defect.

Assessment	Findings
Observe the child for signs of respiratory difficulty (grunting, costal retractions, flaring of the nares, adventitious chest sounds) and hacking cough.	**Clinical Alert** Respiratory difficulties and congested cough may indicate congestive failure or respiratory infection.
Inspect the child's nailbeds for clubbing, lengthening, widening, and splinter hemorrhages (thin, black lines).	**Clinical Alert** Clubbing indicates hypoxia. Splinter hemorrhages indicate emboli.
Examine the anterior chest from an angle. Observe for the symmetry of chest movement, visible pulsations, and diffuse lifts or heaves.	Symmetric chest expansion is normal. In thin children the apical pulse, or point of maximal impulse (PMI), may be seen as a pulsation. **Clinical Alert** Asymmetric chest expansion may signal congestive failure. A systolic heave may indicate right ventricular enlargement.
Palpation	
Using the fingerpads, palpate the anterior chest for the apical pulse or point of maximal impulse (PMI). The location of the PMI is usually felt at the apex of the heart and is found in the fourth intercostal space in children 7 years of age or younger and in the fifth intercostal space in children older than 7 years. The PMI is left of the midclavicular line until 4 years old; midclavicular between 4 and 6 years, and to the right of the line by 7 years.	The apical pulse normally is palpable in infants and young children. **Clinical Alert** A lower, more lateral PMI may indicate cardiac enlargement. An amplified PMI may indicate anemia, fever, or anxiety.
Fingertips are more useful for detecting pulsations, and the ball of the hand (palmar	**Clinical Alert** Rubs are abnormal and should be reported.

Assessment	Findings

surface at the base of the fingers) is useful for detecting vibratory thrills or precordial friction rubs. Thrills feel much like the belly of a purring cat.

Percussion

Percussion is used to estimate heart size by outlining cardiac borders. It is a difficult technique and has limited usefulness in assessing the heart in infants and young children. The location of PMI is a more useful indicator of heart size.

Auscultation

Using both the bell (for low frequency; S_3, S_4 sounds) and the diaphragm (for high frequency; S_1, S_2 sounds), auscultate for heart sounds. Beginning in the second right intercostal space (aortic area), systematically move the stethoscope from the aortic to the pulmonic area (Figure 16-1). S_2 is best heard at the base of the heart (aortic and pulmonic areas). Move down to Erb's point, and then to the tricuspid and mitral areas. S_1 is heard at the beginning of the apical pulse, which facilitates differentiation of S_1 and S_2. Evaluate the sounds for:

Quality (normally S_1 and S_2 are clear and distinct)

S_2 normally loudest in the aortic and pulmonic areas, near the base of the heart.

S_1 and S_2 are equal in intensity at Erb's point.

S_1 is loudest in the mitral and tricuspid areas.

Sinus arrhythmia is a normal variant in which the rate increases with inspiration and decreases with expiration. If unsure whether auscultation suggests sinus arrhythmia or a serious arrhythmia, ask the child to hold the breath. With sinus arrhythmia, holding the breath results in a steady heart rate.

Clinical Alert

S_1 is intensified during fever, exercise, and anemia.

Accentuation of S_1 may also indicate mitral stenosis.

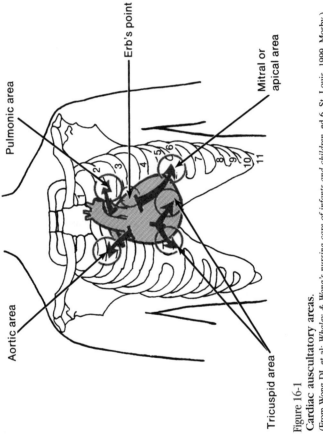

Figure 16-1
Cardiac auscultatory areas.
(From Wong DL et al: *Whaley & Wong's nursing care of infants and children,* ed 6, St. Louis, 1999, Mosby.)

Assessment	Findings
Rate (synchronous with radial pulse)	S_1 that varies in intensity may indicate serious arrhythmia and must be reported.
Intensity (consistent with what would normally be found at each auscultatory point)	
Rhythm (normally regular)	
The child should be helped to assume at least two different positions during auscultation.	
Auscultate for additional sounds, such as S_3 and S_4, which are best assessed with the infant or child lying on the left side. Assess for abnormal sounds such as clicks, murmurs, and precordial friction rubs. Murmurs should be evaluated and documented as to:	S_3 is a normal finding. **Clinical Alert** Innocent or nonpathologic murmurs do not increase over time and do not affect the child's growth. Innocent murmurs are usually systolic (Figure 16-2), medium-pitched, musical, and heard at the second and fourth left interspaces. Innocent murmurs may disappear with change in position.
Location, or auscultatory area in which found	
Timing in the S_1-S_2 cycle	

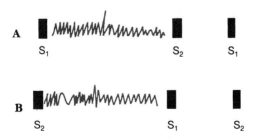

Figure 16-2
Timing of murmurs in S_1-S_2 cycle. **A,** Systolic murmur.
B, Diastolic murmur.

Assessment	Findings
Intensity and whether intensity varies with the child's position. Intensity is usually graded on a six-point scale, with grade 1 being very faint and grade 6 being audible even with the stethoscope off the chest. Grade 3 is considered moderately loud. Pitch Quality (whether murmur is musical, blowing, or swishing) Precordial friction rubs are high-pitched grating or scratching sounds that are unaffected by breathing patterns. Pleural friction rubs stop when children hold their breath.	Organic murmurs are caused by congenital or acquired heart disease. Murmurs occurring before 3 years of age are usually related to congenital defects, and after 3 years to rheumatic heart disease (Table 16-2 provides descriptions of murmurs associated with cardiac defects). Murmurs associated with rheumatic heart disease include those of aortic and mitral stenosis and of aortic and mitral regurgitation. Additional sounds and murmurs must always be described and reported for further evaluation.

Assessment of Vascular System

Assessment of vascular integrity is necessitated by cast application and by other conditions that may impair blood flow. Femoral and dorsal pedal areas should be palpated if cardiac defects are suspected.

Assessment	Findings
Palpate the peripheral arteries for equality, rhythm, and pulse rate. Palpate the radial pulse. The radial pulse is best felt in children older than 2 years of age and who do not evidence spasticity.	Normally pulses are palpable, equal in intensity, and even in rhythm.

Table 16-2 Murmurs Associated with Childhood Cardiac Defects

Defect	Location	Timing	Intensity	Pitch	Quality
Aortic stenosis	Right second interspace (aortic area)	Crescendo effect, occurring between S_1 and S_2	Variable	Medium	Harsh
Pulmonic stenosis	Pulmonic area, third left interspace	Crescendo effect occurring between S_1 and S_2	Variable	Medium	Harsh
Mitral stenosis	Mitral area	Occurs between S_2 and S_1	Variable (Grade 1 to 4); may be accentuated by exercise	Low	Rumbling
Aortic regurgitation	Aortic area	Heard between S_2 and S_1; usually a short period follows S_2 before sound begins	Variable (Grade 1 to 3); most audible when child leans forward and exhales	High; best heard with diaphragm of stethoscope	Blowing May be confused with breath sounds

Continued

Table 16-2 Murmurs Associated with Childhood Cardiac Defects—cont'd

Defect	Location	Timing	Intensity	Pitch	Quality
Mitral regurgitation	Mitral area	Occurs between S_1 and S_2	Variable; unaffected by respiratory cycle	High	Blowing
Ventricular septal defect	Left sternal border, third, fourth, and fifth interspaces	Heard between S_1 and S_2	Very loud	High	Blowing
Patent ductus arteriosus	Second left interspace	Continuous; louder in late systole (just before S_2); obscures S_2; softer in diastole	Loud	Medium	Harsh, machinery like
Tetralogy of Fallot	Second and third left interspaces	Heard between S_1 and S_2	Not well transmitted	—	No distinct characteristics

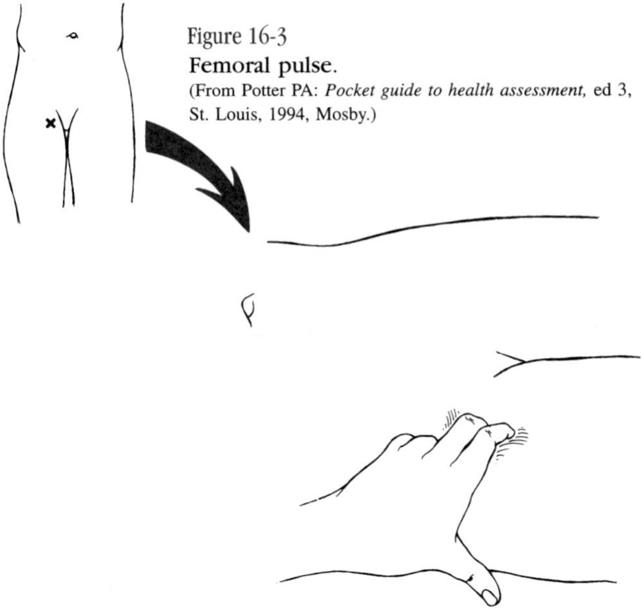

Figure 16-3
Femoral pulse.
(From Potter PA: *Pocket guide to health assessment,* ed 3,
St. Louis, 1994, Mosby.)

Assessment	Findings
Palpate the femoral pulse by applying deep palpation midway between the iliac crest and the symphysis pubis. The child must be in the supine position (Figure 16-3).	**Clinical Alert** Diminution or absence of the femoral pulse may indicate coarctation of the aorta.
Palpate the popliteal pulse by having the child flex the knee (Figure 16-4).	
Palpate the dorsalis pedis pulse along the upper medial aspect of the foot (Figure 16-5).	

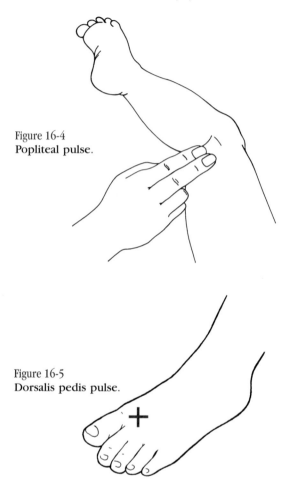

Figure 16-4
Popliteal pulse.

Figure 16-5
Dorsalis pedis pulse.

Related Nursing Diagnoses

Activity intolerance: Related to dyspnea and fatigue secondary to decreased cardiac output.

Imbalanced nutrition, less than body requirements: Related to nausea; fatigue.

Ineffective tissue perfusion: Peripheral secondary to venous congestion; decreased cardiac output.

Anxiety: Related to difficult breathing; situational crisis.

Interrupted family processes: Related to situational crisis; adjustment to chronic disease.

Fear: Related to progressiveness of condition.

Excess fluid volume: Secondary to decreased cardiac output.

Delayed growth and development: Related to activity intolerance; fatigue; social isolation.

Impaired home maintenance: Related to inability to engage in age-appropriate self-care.

Deficient knowledge: Related to diet; drug therapy; signs and symptoms of complications.

Self-care deficit: Related to activity intolerance; fatigue; breathlessness.

Decreased cardiac output: Related to congenital anomalies.

Risk for peripheral neurovascular dysfunction: Related to application of cast.

Risk for impaired skin integrity: Related to fluid retention.

Disturbed sleep pattern: Related to dyspnea secondary to congestive heart failure.

Impaired social interaction: Related to fatigue; limited mobility.

Abdomen

17

Encased within the abdominal cavity are the organs and structures of the genitourinary, gastrointestinal, and hemopoietic systems. Assessment of the abdomen is really a multiple system assessment and commonly follows assessment of the thorax and
lungs.

Lower bowel sounds can be affected by manual manipulation;
thus the order of assessment is inspection, auscultation, percussion,
and palpation. Because it is sometimes performed as part of the
abdominal assessment, assessment of the anus is included in this
chapter.

Rationale

The upper gastrointestinal tract is largely inaccessible to the nurse;
thus examination of the abdomen primarily involves assessment of
lower gastrointestinal and genitourinary structures. Many common
childhood disorders involve the gastrointestinal and genitourinary
systems, and the function of these systems can also be altered by
factors such as surgery, stress, medications, or the hygienic care
that the child receives.

Anatomy and Physiology
Gastrointestinal System

The primary functions of the gastrointestinal tract are the
digestion and absorption of nutrients and water, elimination of
waste products, and secretion of various substances required for
digestion.

The liver, located in the right upper quadrant of the abdomen,
has several important functions, including biosynthesis of protein;
production of blood clotting factors; metabolism of fat, protein,

and carbohydrates; production of bile; metabolism of bilirubin; and detoxification.

A primitive gut develops from the endoderm by the third week of gestation. This developing midgut grows so rapidly that by the fourth week of gestation it is too large for the abdominal cavity. Failure of the midgut to rotate and reenter the abdominal cavity at 10 weeks of gestation can produce a variety of disorders, such as omphalocele, and susceptibility to intussusception and bowel obstruction.

The anus arises from a pit invagination of the skin during embryonic development and is the terminal segment of the anal canal. Normally the anal canal is closed by action of the voluntary external sphincter and involuntary internal sphincter muscles. The canal is well supplied by somatic sensory nerves and is sensitive to touch. Externally it is moist and hairless.

Despite the development of the digestive tract in utero, the exchange of nutrients and waste is the function of the placenta. At birth the gastrointestinal tract is still immature and does not fully mature for the first 2 years. Because of this immaturity, many differences exist between the digestive tract of the infant or child and that of the adult. For example, the muscle tone of the lower esophageal sphincter does not assume adult levels until 1 month of age. This lax sphincter muscle tone explains why young infants frequently regurgitate after feedings. Intestinal peristalsis in children is rapid, with emptying time being 2½ to 3 hours in the newborn infant and 3 to 6 hours in older infants and children. Stomach capacity is 10 to 20 ml (0.3 to 0.6 oz) in the neonate, compared with 10 to 200 ml (0.3 to 7 oz) in the 2-month-old infant, 1500 ml (50 oz) in the 16-year-old adolescent, and 2000 to 3000 ml (89 to 100 oz) in the adult. The stomach is round and lies somewhat horizontally until 2 years of age. The parietal cells of the stomach do not produce adult levels of hydrochloric acid until 6 months. The gastrocolic reflex, or movement of the contents toward the colon, is rapid in young infants, as evidenced by the frequency of stools. The intestine, which underwent rapid growth in utero, undergoes further growth spurts when the child is 1 to 3 years of age and again at 15 to 16 years. After birth the musculature of the anus develops as the infant becomes more upright. The child then becomes able to voluntarily control defecation.

Genitourinary System

The kidneys lie posteriorly within the upper quadrants of the abdomen. The kidneys regulate fluid and electrolyte levels in the body through filtration, reabsorption, and secretion of water and electrolytes. Water is excreted in the form of urine. The bladder, located below the symphysis pubis, collects the urine for elimination.

The development of the kidneys begins early in gestation but is not complete until near the end of the first year of life. Until the epithelial cells of the nephrons assume a mature flat shape, filtration and absorption are poor. The loop of Henle gradually elongates, which increases the infant's ability to concentrate urine, as seen by fewer wet diapers near the first year of life. Increasing bladder capacity also contributes to decreased frequency of voiding. The infant's bladder capacity is 15 to 20 ml (0.5 to 0.7 oz), compared with 600 to 800 ml (20 to 26.7 oz) in the adult. The size of the kidneys varies with size and age. The kidneys of infants and children are relatively large in comparison with those of adults and are more susceptible to trauma because of their size.

Equipment for Assessment of Abdomen

Warm stethoscope
Warm hands
Short fingernails

Preparation

Ask the parent or child about a family history of gastrointestinal or genitourinary tract disorders and about the child's prenatal history (maternal hydramnios is associated with intestinal atresia), mother's lifestyle during pregnancy, and child's growth. Inquire about whether the child had imperforate anus, failure to pass meconium, cleft palate or lip, difficulty in feeding, prolonged jaundice, or abdominal wall disorders (for example, omphalocele or hernia) as a neonate. Ask if the child has or has had problems with feeding such as anorexia, vomiting, or regurgitation or if the child has engaged in fasting or dieting. If the child has had emesis or regurgitation, determine the time of occurrence, frequency, type (Table 17-1), amount, and force (nonprojectile or projectile). Inquire about whether the child has or has had pain (frequency,

Table 17-1   Types of Emesis and Related Findings

Type of Emesis	Related Findings
Undigested formula or food	Rapid expulsion of stomach contents before digestion has occurred.
Yellow; may smell acidic	Contents originated in stomach.
Dark green (bile stained)	Contents originated below the ampulla of Vater.
Dark brown, foul odor	Emesis produced by intestinal obstruction.
Bright red/dark red	Bright red signifies fresh bleeding. Dark red signifies old blood or blood altered by gastric secretions.

intensity, type, location; Table 17-2), itching (location), sleeplessness, swelling, tendency to bruise, thirst, dry mouth, unexplained fever, food allergies, sensitivity to diapers, or alterations in bowel movements or in urinary elimination patterns. If there is a problem with bowel movements, inquire about the frequency, amount, consistency, quality, and color of stool (Table 17-3), use of laxatives and enemas, recent camping trips, and presence of dogs/cats. If there are alterations in the pattern of urinary elimination, determine what they are and when they began. If problems with urination or bowel movements occur in toddlers, explore what these problems mean to parents. In the school-aged child who experiences recurrent abdominal pain, explore possible stressors and responses to stressors. Inquire about body piercings, tatoos, and environmental factors such as daycare, crowded living conditions, and sharing of utensils and other personal items.

It is important that the child be relaxed during abdominal examination, particularly during palpation. Flexing the child's head or hips helps relax abdominal muscles. Asking the child to "suck in" or "puff out" the abdomen helps assess the degree of discomfort present before deeper probing. Flexing the child's knees permits greater visibility of the anal area. Talking and playing with the child also assists in examination. Most children are ticklish, so briefly place a hand flat on the abdomen before beginning the examination. A very ticklish child can be assisted by placing the child's hand over the nurse's during palpation.

Text continued on p. 202

Table 17-2 Characteristics and Common Etiologies of Acute Abdominal Pain in Children

Location	Characteristics	Age-Group	Possible Etiology	Related Factors	Associated Symptoms
Lower abdominal, flank	Severe, colicky	Adolescent	Urolithiasis	• Hypercalciuria • Urinary tract infection	• Restlessness • Dysuria
Lower abdominal, especially suprapubic	Constant	Any	Cystitis	• Bubble baths • Tight jeans • Nylon panties • Sexual activity	• Urinary frequency • Dysuria
Lower abdominal		Any	Obstruction	• Adhesions related to surgery • Ingestion of hairballs or trichobezoars • Developmental or psychological problems	• Frequent tinkling sounds (early obstruction) or high-pitched rumbles • Diminished bowel sounds (late obstruction) • Absence of bowel sounds (total obstruction)
Lower abdomen	Acute or chronic, crampy	Older school-aged or adolescent	Ulcerative colitis	• Infection • Dietary habits • Familial tendency	• Diarrhea • Blood in stools • Growth failure

Location	Timing	Age	Condition	History	Signs
Bilateral, lower abdomen	Constant	Adolescent	Pelvic inflammatory disease	• Multiple sex partners • Alcohol/drug use • Begin during or within week of menses	• Guarding upon palpation • Fever • Pain with movement • Walks slightly bent over and tends to hold abdomen
	Constant	Adolescent	Endometriosis	• Menses	• Morning vomiting
	Constant, crampy	Adolescent	Ectopic pregnancy	• Amenorrhea	
	Constant, crampy	Any	Constipation	• Spinal injury • Meningomyelocele • Use of anticholinergics, laxatives • Eating disorders	• Lack of stooling • Bloating • Presence of a mass
Nonspecific	Chronic	School-age adolescent	Psychogenic	• Abuse • Depression • Eating disorders • Minor adjustment problems	• Pain may interfere with stressful activities but not with pleasurable ones • May be associated with specific situations • Eyes remain closed during palpation

Continued

Table 17-2 Characteristics and Common Etiologies of Acute Abdominal Pain in Children—cont'd

Location	Characteristics	Age-Group	Possible Etiology	Related Factors	Associated Symptoms
Generalized		Any	Streptococcal pharyngitis	• Infection	• Erythematous pharynx • Fever • Pain
Periumbilical	Crampy	Older school-aged or adolescent	Crohn's disease	• Infection • Dietary habits • Familial tendency	• Weight loss • Anorexia • Poor growth • Borborygmi • Abdominal distention
	Colicky	Any	Lactose intolerance	• Symptoms occur after milk ingestion • Cultural and hereditary factors	• Watery stools
	Crampy	Any	Gastroenteritis	• Infection	• Vomiting • Diarrhea • Dehydration • Fever
	Constant, upon deep inspiration	Any	Pneumonia	• Infection • Aspiration	• Cough • Fever • Malaise • Rales

	Colicky	Any	Diabetic ketoacidosis	• Absent or inadequate supply of insulin

- Polydipsia
- Polyuria
- Headache
- Kussmaul respirations

Periumbilical (nontender) in early stages followed by generalized and then right lower quadrant pain (tender)	Constant, increasing	Preschool, school-aged, adolescent	Appendicitis	• Hardened fecal material • Parasites • Foreign bodies

- Anorexia
- Vomiting
- Fever
- Leukocytosis
- Rebound tenderness
- Flex hip on affected side

Epigastric	Dull ache	Adolescent	Esophagitis	• Self-induced vomiting

- Vomiting

			Hepatitis	• Exchange of blood or any bodily fluid or secretion • Fecal-oral transmission

- Nausea and vomiting
- Fever
- Anorexia
- Pruritus
- Jaundice

Continued

Table 17-2   Characteristics and Common Etiologies of Acute Abdominal Pain in Children—cont'd

Location	Characteristics	Age-Group	Possible Etiology	Related Factors	Associated Symptoms
Epigastric—cont'd	Sharp, constant, sudden	Adolescent	Pancreatitis	• Alcohol ingestion • Lying supine may aggravate	
	Stabbing, burning, radiates to back	Adolescent	Duodenal ulcer	• Blood group (O) • Familial tendency • Ulcerogenic drugs • Alcohol • Smoking • Bacterium *H. pylori* • *Stress*	• Hematemesis • Melena • Anemia • Poor eating habits
Epigastric area, right upper quadrant, shoulder, right scapula	May be dull, crampy, acute, or gradual	Adolescent more common than children	Cholecystitis	• Oral contraceptive use • Ingestion of fatty or acidic foods	• Nausea • Bloating • Guarding upon palpation

Table 17-3   Types of Stools and Related Findings

Type of Stool	Related Findings
Soft or liquid	Indicative of breast-feeding.
Light yellow, pasty. Soft or pasty green	Common in formula-fed babies. Stool has been exposed to air for some time, and oxidation has occurred.
Watery, pale	Associated with celiac disease.
Liquid or watery green	Diarrhea. Indicative of infectious disorders, inflammatory bowel disease, chemotherapy, Hirschsprung's disease, or laxative use.
Grossly bloody diarrhea	May be indicative of ulcerative colitis or infectious dysenteries.
Black	May indicate that the child is receiving iron or bismuth preparations or has gastric or duodenal bleeding.
Gray or clay colored	Biliary atresia may be present.
Undigested food in stool	Common in infants who are unable to completely digest foods, such as corn and carrots.
Currant jelly stool (blood and mucus)	Indicative of intussusception, Meckel's diverticulum. Found with Henoch-Schönlein purpura.
Ribbon-like	Indicative of Hirschsprung's disease.
Frothy, foul smelling	Indicative of cystic fibrosis.
Firm, hard stool	Associated with diet, inadequate fluid or fiber intake, encopresis, obstructive disorders, irritable bowel syndrome, chemotherapy, medications; overly rigid toilet training.

Assessment of Abdomen

Assessment	Findings
Inspection	
Inspect the contour of the abdomen while the infant or child is standing and while he or she is lying supine.	A pot-bellied or prominent abdomen is normal until puberty, related to lordosis of the spine. The abdomen appears flat when the child is supine. **Clinical Alert** An especially protuberant abdomen may suggest fluid retention, tumor, organomegaly (enlarged organ), or ascites. A large abdomen, with thin limbs and wasted buttocks, suggests severe malnutrition and may be seen in children with celiac disease or cystic fibrosis. A depressed abdomen is indicative of dehydration or high abdominal obstruction. A midline protrusion from the xiphoid process to the umbilicus or the symphysis pubis indicates diastasis recti abdominis.
Inspect the color and condition of the skin of the abdomen. Note the presence of scars, ecchymoses, and stomas or pouches.	**Clinical Alert** Yellowish coloration may suggest jaundice. Jaundice is found with hepatitis, cirrhosis, gallbladder disease. Silver lines (striae) indicate obesity or fluid retention. Scars may indicate previous surgery. Ecchymoses of soft tissue areas can indicate abuse. Distended veins indicate abdominal or vascular obstruction or distention.

Assessment	Findings
Inspect the abdomen for movement by standing at eye level to the abdomen.	**Clinical Alert**
	Visible peristaltic waves nearly always indicate intestinal obstruction, and in the infant younger than 2 months indicate pyloric stenosis. If an infant younger than 2 months is fed, the peristaltic waves become larger and more frequent if stenosis is present.
	Failure of the abdomen and thorax to move synchronously may indicate peritonitis (if the abdomen does not move) or pulmonary disease (if the thorax does not move).
Inspect the umbilicus for color, discharge, odor, inflammation, and herniation.	**Clinical Alert**
	A bluish umbilicus indicates intraabdominal hemorrhage.
	A nodular umbilicus indicates tumor.
	Protrusion of the umbilicus indicates herniation. Umbilical hernias protrude more noticeably with crying and coughing. Palpate the umbilicus to estimate the size of the opening.
	Drainage from the umbilicus may indicate infection or a patent urachus.

Auscultation

Auscultate for bowel sounds by pressing both the bell and the diaphragm of the stethoscope *firmly* against the abdomen. Listen in all four quadrants (Figure 17-1) and count the bowel sounds in each quadrant for 1 full minute. Before	Normal bowel sounds occur every 10 to 30 seconds and are heard as gurgles, clicks, and growls.
	Clinical Alert
	High-pitched tinkling sounds indicate diarrhea, gastroenteritis, or obstruction.

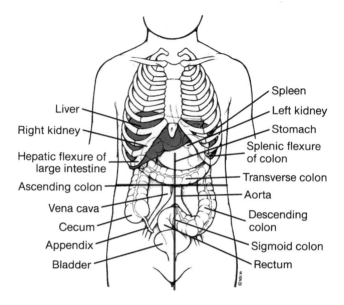

Figure 17-1
Anatomic landmarks of abdomen.
(From Whaley LF, Wong DL: *Nursing care of infants and children,* ed 4,
St. Louis, 1991, Mosby.)

Assessment	Findings
deciding that bowel sounds are absent, the nurse must listen for a minimum of 5 minutes in each area where sounds are not heard. Bowel sounds can be stimulated, if present, by stroking the abdomen with a fingernail.	Absence of bowel sounds may indicate peritonitis or paralytic ileus.

Percussion

Using indirect percussion, systematically percuss all areas of the abdomen.	Dullness or flatness is normally found along the right costal margin (see Figure 17-1) and 1 to 3 cm (0.4 to 1.4 in) below the costal margin of the liver.

Assessment	Findings
	Dullness above the symphysis pubis may indicate a full bladder in a young child and is normal.
	Tympany is normally heard throughout the rest of the abdomen.
	Clinical Alert
	Areas of unexpected dullness or flatness may indicate large masses of feces.
	If liver dullness extends lower than expected, an enlarged liver may be suspected.

Palpation

If the child complains of pain in an abdominal area, palpate that area last.

Assessment	Findings
Using superficial palpation, assess the abdomen for tenderness, superficial lesions, muscle tone, turgor (pinch the skin into a fold), and cutaneous hyperesthesia (pick up a fold of skin but do not pinch). Superficial palpation is performed by placing the hand on the abdomen and applying light pressure with the fingertips. Note areas of tenderness. *Visceral* pain, arising from organs, is dull and poorly localized. *Somatic* pain, arising from the walls and the linings of the abdominal cavity, is sharp and well defined. Do not ask, "Does this hurt?" The child, eager to please, may say yes. A pain measurement scale may help	**Clinical Alert**
	A child's withdrawal or tense facial expression may indicate apprehension, pain, or nausea.
	Pain on picking up a fold of abdominal skin indicates cutaneous hyperesthesia, which may be found with peritonitis.

Assessment	Findings

children to rate pain more specifically and to differentiate between pain and fear. During palpation, observe if the child's eyes are closed; a child with genuine pain will tend to watch the palpating hand closely.

Perform deep palpation, either by placing one hand on top of the other or by supporting posterior structures with one hand while palpating anterior structures with the other. Palpate from the lower quadrants upward so that an enlarged liver can be detected.

Discomfort in the epigastrium on deep palpation is related to pressure over the aorta.

The spleen tip may be palpated 1 to 2 cm (0.4 to 0.8 in) below the left costal margin during inspiration in infants and young children and is felt as a soft, thumb-shaped object.

The liver may be palpated below the right costal margin during inspiration in infants and young children. The liver edge is firm and smooth.

Kidneys are rarely palpable except in neonates.

The sigmoid colon may be palpable as a tender sausage-shaped mass in the left lower quadrant. The cecum may be palpated as a soft mass in the right lower quadrant.

Clinical Alert

Tenderness in the lower quadrants may indicate feces, gastroenteritis, pelvic infection, or tumor.

Tenderness in the left upper quadrant may indicate splenic enlargement or intussusception.

Assessment	Findings
	An enlarged spleen indicates infection or blood disease.
	Tenderness in the right upper quadrant may be related to hepatitis or an enlarged liver.
	Tenderness in the right lower quadrant or around the umbilicus may indicate appendicitis. *Rebound tenderness* indicates appendicitis and may be elicited by applying pressure distal to where the child states there is pain. Pain is experienced in the original area of tenderness when pressure is *released.*
	An enlarged liver is found with infection, blood dycrasias, and sickle cell anemia.
	Enlarged kidneys may indicate tumor or hydronephrosis.
	Intestinal masses may indicate tumors or stool.
	A distended bladder may be palpable above the symphysis pubis.
Further assess for peritoneal irritation by performing the psoas muscle test. This test can be performed in a cooperative older child if the nurse is assessing for appendicitis. Have the child flex the right leg at the hip and knee while you apply downward pressure. Normally, no pain is felt.	**Clinical Alert** Pain suggests appendicitis.
Palpate for an inguinal hernia by sliding the little finger into the external inguinal canal at the base of the scrotum and	**Clinical Alert** Report the presence of inguinal hernia. An inguinal hernia is felt as a bulge when the child

Assessment	Findings
ask the child to cough. If the child is young, have child laugh or blow up a balloon.	laughs or cries. Inguinal hernia is more common in boys.
Palpate for a femoral hernia by locating the femoral pulse. Place the index finger on the pulse and the middle or ring finger medially against the skin. The ring finger is over the area where the herniation occurs.	**Clinical Alert** Report the presence of femoral hernia. A femoral hernia is felt or seen as a small anterior mass. Femoral hernia is more commonly found in girls.

Assessment of Anal Area

Assessment	Findings
With the child prone, inspect the buttocks and thighs. Examine the skin around the anal area for redness and rash.	**Clinical Alert** Asymmetry of the buttocks and thigh folds indicates congenital hip dysplasia. Redness and rash may indicate inadequate cleaning after bowel movements, infrequent changing of diapers, or irritation from diarrhea.
Examine the anus for marks, fissures (tears in the mucosa), hemorrhoids (dark protrusions), prolapse (moist tube-like protrusion), polyps (bright red protrusions), and skin tags.	The anus usually appears moist and hairless. **Clinical Alert** Scratch marks may indicate itching, which can indicate pinworm infestation. Fissures may indicate passage of hard stools. Defecation may be accompanied by bleeding if fissures are present. Bleeding can also accompany polyps, intussusception, gastric and peptic ulcers, esophageal varices, ulcerative colitis, infectious diseases, and Meckel's diverticulum.

Assessment	Findings
	Rectal prolapse indicates difficult defecation and often accompanies untreated cystic fibrosis.
	Skin tags can indicate polyps and are usually benign.
	Lacerations and bruises of anus may indicate abuse.
Stroke the anal area to elicit the anal reflex.	The anus should contract quickly.
	Clinical Alert
	A slow reflex may indicate a disorder of the pyramidal tract.

Related Nursing Diagnoses

Anxiety: Related to knowledge deficit; discomfort.

Constipation: Related to altered bowel motility; diet.

Diarrhea: Related to altered bowel motility; diet; use of laxatives.

Impaired comfort: Pain related to altered bowel motility; bowel distention; bladder distention; altered stomach function; loss of skin integrity; pruritus; stress; injury.

Interrupted family processes: Related to skill or knowledge deficit; stress.

Deficient fluid volume: Related to excess fluid loss; limited intake; increased metabolic rate.

Excess fluid volume: Secondary to liver disorders; renal disorders.

Ineffective health maintenance: Related to knowledge deficit; self-esteem; lifestyle choices.

Deficient knowledge: Related to disease process; dietary alterations; hygienic needs; dietary needs.

Impaired parenting: Related to skill deficit.

Impaired skin integrity: Related to pruritus; knowledge deficit; incontinence (urine or feces).

Impaired urinary elimination, alterations in patterns of: Related to inflammation; infection; retention; artificial drainage system.

Lymphatic System

18

The lymphatic system includes the lymph nodes, spleen, thymus, and bone marrow. The superficial lymph nodes and the spleen are accessible for assessment and are discussed in this chapter. Assessment of the lymphatic system is often integrated with assessment of the neck, breast, and abdomen.

Rationale

The most common causes of visible lymphoid activity are infection and neoplasms. Infection is the most common cause of lumps in children's necks. An understanding of which areas are drained by the nodes is useful in further assessment of present or past infections. Detection of enlarged nodes and an enlarged spleen can be critical to the early diagnosis and treatment of serious disorders.

Anatomy and Physiology

The lymphoid system is a system of lymph fluid, collecting ducts, and tissues. Although the specific functions of lymphoid tissue are still not fully understood, the system is thought to play an important role in the production of lymphocytes and antibodies and in phagocytosis. The system also transports lymph fluids, microorganisms, and protein back to the cardiovascular system and absorbs fat and fat-soluble substances from the intestine.

Lymph enters open-ended ducts called *capillaries.* The capillaries form larger collecting ducts, which drain into tissue centers or nodes. Lymph from the nodes eventually drains into the venous system by way of even larger ducts.

Lymph nodes, the most numerous element in the lymphatic system, rarely occur singly, but usually in chains or clusters. The lymph nodes that are closer to the center of the body are usually smaller; thus cervical nodes are larger than axillary nodes. The spleen is composed of lymphoid and reticuloendothelial cells. It is found under the ribs in the upper left quadrant of the abdomen. The amount of lymphoid tissue and the size of the lymph nodes vary with age. Infants have a small amount of palpable lymphatic tissue, which gradually increases until middle childhood, when the volume of lymphatic tissue reaches its peak. By mid-adolescence the volume of lymphatic tissue begins to diminish, until it reaches the adult level of 2% to 3% of total body weight. Children are more likely to develop generalized adenopathy in response to disease, and even mild infections result in swollen nodes or "swollen glands."

Equipment for Assessment of Lymphatic System

Ruler

Preparation

Inquire about recent contacts with persons with infectious diseases. Ask if the child has been experiencing weakness, easy fatigability, fever, bruising, or chronic or recurrent infection. Ask if there is a family history of blood disorders or cancer.

Assessment of Lymph Nodes

Assessment	Findings
Using the distal portion of the fingers and gentle but firm circular motions, palpate the head, neck, axillae, and groin to detect enlarged lymph nodes (Figure 18-1). Note the color, size, location, mobility, temperature, consistency, and tenderness of enlarged nodes. Tender nodes should be assessed last. Measure enlarged nodes.	Small (less than 1 cm, or ½ in), movable, nontender nodes are normal in young children. **Clinical Alert** Nodes that are enlarged because of infection are firm, warm, fluctuant, and movable, and their borders are diffuse. Redness may overlie nodes that are enlarged because of infection.

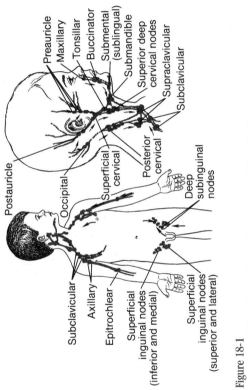

Figure 18-1
Location of lymph nodes and direction of lymph flow.
(From Wong DL et al: *Whaley & Wong's nursing care of infants and children*, ed 6, St. Louis, 1999, Mosby.)

Assessment	Findings
To palpate nodes in the areas anterior and posterior to the sternocleidomastoid muscle, move the fingertips against the muscle.	Enlargement of preauricular nodes commonly suggests eye infection.
To palpate nodes in the head and neck, have the child flex the head forward or bend toward the side being examined.	Enlargement of the preauricular, mastoid, and deep cervical nodes may indicate infection of the ear.
To palpate nodes in the axillae, roll the tissues against the chest wall and muscles of the axillae. Have the child hold the arms in a relaxed, slightly abducted position at the sides.	Enlargement of nodes in the jaw area may signify infections of the tongue or mouth.
To palpate nodes in the inguinal area, place the child supine.	Enlargement of nodes in the supraclavicular region often indicates metastases from the lungs or abdominal structures.
	Bilateral lymph node enlargement may indicate infectious nucleosis.
	Nodes enlarged as a result of cancer are usually nontender, fixed, hard, of variable size, and matted. No discoloration is present.
	Enlarged nodes may also indicate metabolic disorders, hypersensitivity reactions, and primary hematopoietic disorders.

Assessment of Spleen

Assessment	Findings
With the child supine, place one hand under the child's back and the other hand on the left upper quadrant of the child's abdomen. Ask the child to "Suck in your breath." The spleen tip can be felt during inspiration on deep palpation.	The spleen can be palpated 1 to 2 cm (0.4 to 0.8 in) below the left costal margin in infants and children. **Clinical Alert** A spleen that extends more than 2 cm (0.8 in) below the costal margin may indicate leukemia, thalassemia major, sickle cell anemia, or infectious mononucleosis.

Related Nursing Diagnoses

Activity intolerance: Related to weakness; fatigue.

Compromised family coping: Related to situational crisis; knowledge deficit.

Hyperthermia: Related to infection.

Injury, potential for: Related to presence of infective organisms.

Imbalanced nutrition: Less than body requirements related to increased metabolism.

Reproductive System 19

Assessment of the reproductive system in infants and children includes inspection of the external genitalia. Examination of internal genitalia is performed by nurses specially prepared in this skill.

Rationale

Examination of the external genitalia enables screening for common disorders that arise from prenatal development and influences. Examination enables the nurse to detect infections that require further evaluation. Assessment of the reproductive system often provides a beginning point for teaching and discussion related to sexuality and hygiene.

Anatomy and Physiology
Female Genitalia

The female genitalia includes the external and internal sex organs. The external sex organs, or vulva, include the mons pubis, a fatty pad overlying the symphysis pubis (Figure 19-1); the labia majora, rounded folds of adipose tissue extending down and back from the mons pubis; the labia minora, two thinner folds of skin medial to the labia majora, which, following prominence in the newborn period, atrophy to become nearly invisible until adolescence; and the clitoris, an erectile body situated at the anterior end of the labia minora. The labia minora are homologous to the male scrotum, and the clitoris to the male penis. Underlying the labia minora is a boat-shaped area termed the *vestibule*. At the posterior end of the vestibule is the vaginal opening, or introitus, which may be partially obscured by the hymen, a vascular mucous membrane. The perineum is the area between the vaginal opening and the anus. The urethral opening, or urinary meatus, lies between the vaginal opening and the clitoris. On either side of the urethral opening can be seen Skene's glands, or the paraurethral ducts. Bartholin's glands, which secrete lubricating fluid during intercourse, are situated on either side of the vaginal opening, but the openings to the glands usually cannot be seen.

The vagina is a hollow tube extending upward and backward between the urethra and the rectum. The cervix joins the vagina, which has a slitlike opening, termed the *external os,* that provides an opening between the uterus and the endocervical canal. The uterus is a muscular pear-shaped organ suspended above the bladder. In the prepubescent girl the uterus is 2.5 to 3.5 cm (1 to 1.5 in) long, compared with 6 to 8 cm (2.4 to 3.2 in) in the mature woman. The uterine, or fallopian, tubes extend from the uterus to the ovaries and produce a passageway in which ova and sperm meet.

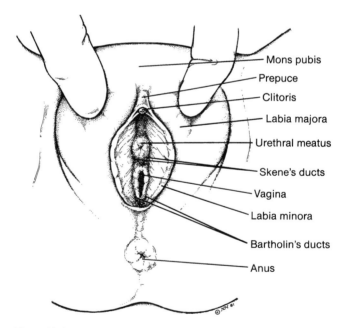

Figure 19-1
External female genitalia.
(From Whaley LF, Wong DL: *Nursing care of infants and children,* ed 4, St. Louis, 1991, Mosby.)

Male Genitalia

The external male genitalia includes the penis and scrotum. The penis consists of a shaft and a glans (Figure 19-2). The shaft is formed primarily of erectile tissue. The glans is a cone-shaped structure at the end of the penis and contains both erectile and sensory tissue. The corona is the crownlike area where the glans arises from the shaft. A loose fold of skin, termed the *prepuce* or foreskin, overlies the glans. This skin is removed during circumcision. The urethra is within the penile shaft, with the slitlike urethral meatus located slightly centrally at the tip of the glans.

The scrotum is a loose, wrinkled sac located at the base of the penis. The scrotum has two compartments, each of which contains a testis, epididymis, and parts of the vas deferens. The testes, epididymis, and vas deferens are considered internal male sex organs.

The testes are ovoid and somewhat rubbery. The testes in the infant are 1.5 cm (0.6 in) long. Testicular length remains virtually unchanged until puberty, when the testes gradually enlarge to the adult length of 4 to 5 cm (1.6 to 2 in). The left testis lies slightly lower than the right. Primary functions of the testis are sperm and hormone production. During ejaculation, sperm drains into the

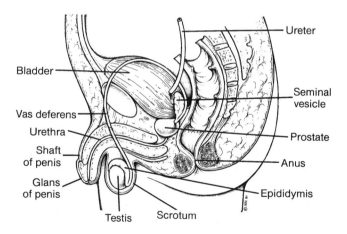

Figure 19-2
Male genitalia.
(From Whaley LF, Wong DL: *Nursing care of infants and children,* ed 4, St. Louis, 1991, Mosby.)

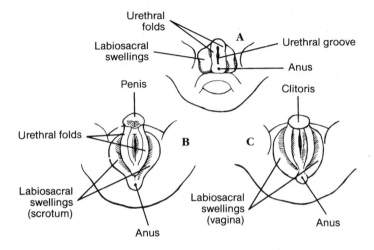

Figure 19-3
Initial stages in embryonic genital development. **A,** Undifferentiated stage. **B,** Initial differentiation of external genitalia in male embryo. **C,** Initial differentiation of external genitalia in female embryo.

epididymis, and then into the vas deferens before passing into the urethra.

The genetic sex type of the embryo begins during cell division, when X and Y chromosomes are distributed. Initially, internal and external genitalia are not differentiated (Figure 19-3, *A*). External differentiation begins by about the seventh week of gestation. Under the influence of androgens, enlargement and fusion of primitive urogenital structures occurs and male genitalia are formed (Figure 19-3, *B*). The testes descend from the abdominal cavity at between 7 and 9 months of gestation. If the tube that precedes their descent fails to close, an indirect inguinal hernia is produced.

The male reproductive system remains unchanged until maturity. Testicular enlargement is a visible sign of sexual maturation, which may begin by 10 years of age. Accompanying the initial increase in testicular size are a coarsening, reddening, and wrinkling of the scrotal sacs and the growth of a few pubic hairs (the child has no pubic hair). Height and weight increase, and hair growth appears on the face about 2 years after the appearance of pubic hair. During further development the penis enlarges, the voice changes, and body odor appears. The genital skin continues to pigment and the external sex organs continue to enlarge until full maturation is reached. At maturity pubic hair covers the symphysis pubis and medial aspects of the thighs. Reproductive capability accompanies sexual maturity, which is accomplished between 14 and 18 years of age.

In the embryo, development of female genitalia involves shrinkage and minimal fusion of primitive urogenital structures (Figure 19-3, *C*). Primordial follicles are formed during the sixth month of gestation, but must wait until puberty for further development. Breast development is usually the first sign of sexual maturation, although growth of pubic hair may precede breast enlargement. The initial pubic hair, located at the sides of the labia, is fine. Gradually the hair coarsens and covers the sides of the labia and the perianal area at full maturation. Internal and external sex organs enlarge. The onset of menstruation provides observable evidence of reproductive maturation (Figure 19-4).

Equipment for Assessment of Reproductive System

Glove for pelvic examination
Drape
Speculum

Preparation

A casual, matter-of-fact approach facilitates examination of the reproductive system. Much of the examination can be accomplished during assessment of the abdomen and anus in the infant and younger child. Inform parents (if appropriate) and child of results of the finding as the assessment progresses because this helps relieve anxiety. A child other than an infant should be adequately covered at all times with clothing or a drape and alternative positions for examination, such as semisitting, may be more comfortable. An adolescent should be given the option of having a supportive person, such as a friend present during examination. It is important to ensure privacy and confidentiality and if a parent is present, it must be made clear the adolescent is

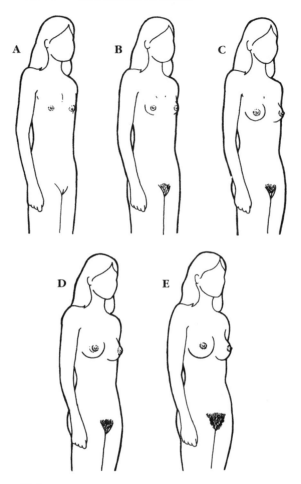

Figure 19-4

Tanner stages in development of female breasts and female pubic hair. **A,** Prepubescent. Papilla elevates. No pubic hair. **B,** Breast bud stage. Breast and papilla elevated as a small mound. Areola enlarges. Sparse long, straight pubic hair. **C,** Breast and areola enlarge further. Heavier, coarser pubic hair. **D,** Areola and papilla project from breast. Pubic hair similar to that in adult but covers smaller area. **E,** Mature form. Papilla elevates but areola recedes into breast. Pubic hair is adultlike distribution and quantity.

the patient by directing questions at him or her. It is important to recognize that children and parents from some cultures (for example, Hispanic) are particularly modest and may require additional assistance to become comfortable.

The first pelvic examination is usually performed when the female child is 18 to 21 years old or as soon as she becomes sexually active, when there is a history of trauma or abuse, when there is vaginal discharge, menorrhagia, primary amenorrhea, secondary amenorrhea for more than 3 months, abdominal pain, or at the adolescent's request. Adolescents at high risk (sexual intercourse before 18 years, multiple partners, intercourse without a condom, partners with history of intercourse, smoking, sexually transmitted diseases, and absence of three consecutive, negative Pap smears) should be screened yearly.

Inquire whether the female child has or has had itching, pain on urination, abdominal pain, or vaginal discharge. If the girl is older, inquire whether menses have commenced, the date of the last menstrual period, length of cycle, amount of flow, if the adolescent knows how to or is practicing breast self-examination, dietary and exercise regimen, and type of contraception used (if sexually active), number of sexual partners, and experiences with sexual abuse and rape. Inquire about family history of breast cancer and ovarian cancer. If the child has missed three consecutive menses, inquire about eating habits.

Inquire whether the male child has or has had decreased urination, forced urination, a strong urinary stream, or pain on voiding, discharge or drip from the penis, and if sexually active, if using a condom. Inquire if adolescent knows how or is practicing testicular self-examination.

Assessment of Female Breasts

Assessment is accomplished with the adolescent sitting with arms at her sides. Because the adolescent must disrobe to the waist, ensure that the room is warm. Privacy is essential. Tell the adolescent that you are going to examine her breasts. A gentle matter-of-fact approach assists in putting her at ease. If the adolescent is unfamiliar with breast self-examination, this is a good opportunity to explain what is being done and to encourage her to imitate the examination maneuvers. Adolescents may be too embarrassed to touch their breasts, and the nurse's approach should vary with the patient's degree of psychologic comfort.

Assessment	Findings
Inspect the breasts. Note their size, contour, symmetry, and color while the child or adolescent is sitting, bare to the waist, and arms at side.	Contour and size of the breasts and changes in the areola indicate sexual maturity. Some difference in size of the breasts is usually normal.
	One breast may develop before the other, and the adolescent may need reassurance that this is normal.
	Clinical Alert
	Breast development before 8 years of age may be normal but requires careful assessment.
	Delayed breast development (none by age 13 years) should be evaluated along with the development of secondary sexual characteristics.
	Dimpling and alterations in the contour of the breast may indicate cancer.
	Redness may signal infection.
Inspect the nipple and areola. Note their color, size, shape, and the presence and color of any discharge.	The color, size, and shape of the nipple and areola provide information about sexual maturity.
	Clinical Alert
	Flattening of the nipple in a more mature adolescent or edema of the nipple or areola may indicate the presence of cancer.
	Discharge is an abnormal finding and may be due to a number of hormonal and pharmacologic causes. It should, however, be referred to a physician.

Assessment	Findings
Have the adolescent place her arms above her head, and then on her hips. These maneuvers help accentuate dimpling or retraction that may be missed. Note axilla hair.	African American girls develop axillary hair sooner than Caucasian counterparts (Tanner stages are based on studies of white, English girls) and sometimes before pubic hair. Asian adolescents tend to have finer and sparser hair.
Palpate the breast tissue with the patient supine and with her hands behind her neck. If breasts are large, place a pillow under the patient's shoulder on the side that is to be examined. This distributes the breast tissue more evenly. Use the pads of the fingers flat on the breast to gently compress the tissue against the chest wall. Systematically palpate the entire breast, including the periphery, areola, nipple, and tail using a pattern such as parallel lines, concentric circles, or consecutive clock times. During palpation note consistency of tissues and areas of tenderness.	Normal young breast tissue has firm elasticity. The stimulation of examination may cause erection of the nipple and wrinkling of the areola. **Clinical Alert** Fixed, hard nodules with unclear borders may indicate cancer.
Palpate abnormal masses and note their location (by quadrant or clock), size (in centimeters or inches), shape (round, discoid, irregular), consistency (soft, firm, hard), tenderness, mobility, discreteness (well-circumscribed or not).	**Clinical Alert** Fixed, hard, irregular, and poorly circumscribed nodules may suggest cancer. Mobile, nontender, round or disclike, well-delineated nodules may indicate fibroadenoma.

Assessment of Female Genitalia

Assessment is best accomplished with the child supine or semi-reclining (if a young child, examination can be performed with child semireclining in the parent's lap). Encouraging the child to keep her heels together provides distraction. Before beginning a pelvic examination, have the adolescent empty her bladder.

Assessment	Findings
Inspect the mons pubis for hair. Note color, quality, quantity, and distribution of hair, if present.	Soft, downy hair along the labia majora signals early sexual maturation. In the mature woman, pubic hair forms an inverted triangle.
Inspect the labia majora and labia minora for size, color, skin integrity, masses, and lesions.	Labia should appear pink and moist. **Clinical Alert** Redness and swelling of labia may indicate infection, masturbation, or sexual abuse. Fusion of labia may indicate male scrotum. Labial adhesions may be seen in infants. Blisters, pimples, chancres, and warts may indicate venereal disease. Venereal disease in the young child is a sign of sexual abuse. Urogenital abnormalities are found in infants born to mothers who used cocaine prenatally.
Note the size of the clitoris.	**Clinical Alert** A clitoris larger than normal may indicate labioscrotal fusion. In some cultures, female circumcision is practiced, which can produce extensive scarring and adhesions.

Assessment	Findings
Palpate for Skene's and Bartholin's glands.	Skene's and Bartholin's glands are normally not palpable.
Inspect urethral and vaginal openings for edema, redness, and discharge.	A small amount of clear, mucousy discharge is normal.
	Clinical Alert
	If Bartholin's or Skene's glands are palpable, infection or cysts may be present.
	Clinical Alert
	Redness of the urethra may indicate urethritis.
	Hymen tears, enlarged hymenal opening, irregular or thickened hymenal edges, and attenuation of hymenal tissue may indicate abuse.
	Redness and foul-smelling discharge from the vagina may indicate a foreign body, infection, sexual abuse, or pinworms.
	A white, cheesy discharge from the vagina indicates a candidal infection.
	Refer the child for further examination if a vaginal opening cannot be seen.
Initiate the speculum examination in the adolescent after inspection of external structures. Use a plastic or metal speculum that has been lubricated and warmed with warm water. Usually the narrow Pederson speculum is used.	
Initiate the bimanual examination following the speculum examination. Inability to feel ovaries is not unusual, especially if the adolescent is overweight.	

Assessment of Male Genitalia

Assessment	Findings
Inspect the penis for size, color, skin integrity, masses, and lesions. Note whether the child is circumcised. If un-circumcised and older than 3 years of age, attempt to retract the foreskin. Do not forcibly attempt to retract the foreskin.	An obese child may appear to have a small penis because of overlying skin folds. The foreskin is normally adher-ent in children younger than 3 years. **Clinical Alert** A penis that is large in relation to the child's stage of devel-opment may suggest preco-cious puberty or testicular cancer. An abnormally small penis may indicate a clitoris. A round, dark red, painless sore is a syphilitic chancre and should be reported. Condyloma acuminatum, or warts, is a venereal disease and may indicate sexual ac-tivity in an adolescent or sexual abuse in a young child. A foreskin that cannot be easily retracted in a child older than 3 years may indicate phimosis.
Inspect the urinary meatus for shape, placement, discharge, and ulceration. If possible, note the strength and steadi-ness of the urinary stream.	The urinary meatus is normally *slightly* ventral at the tip of the penis and slitlike. **Clinical Alert** A urinary meatus that is ventral is called *hypospadias.* A meatus that is dorsal is called *epispadias.* A round meatus may be indica-tive of meatal stenosis related to repeated infections.

Assessment	Findings
Inspect the quality, quantity, and distribution of pubic hair. Inspect the base of the penis for scratches and inflammation. Inspect the scrotum for color, size, symmetry, edema, masses, and lesions. Palpate the testes by holding a finger over the inguinal canal while palpating the scrotal sac. Cold, touch, exercise, and stimulation cause the testes to ascend higher into the pelvic cavity. This can be prevented by palpating the inguinal canal or by having the child sit tailor fashion.	A prepubertal boy normally does not have pubic hair (Figure 19-5). The left testis is lower than the right. A testis should be present in each sac, freely movable, smooth, equal in size, and about 1.5 cm (0.8 in) until puberty. **Clinical Alert** The absence of a testis in the scrotal sac may indicate temporary ascent of the testis into the pelvic cavity or an undescended testicle. Reassess. If testes still cannot be felt, refer the child if older than 3 years. Before 3 years the testicle may descend without intervention. If both testes are undescended, this may indicate pseudohermaphroditism, especially if hypospadias or a small penis is also present. Delayed pubertal changes may indicate chronic illness or abnormalities in the anterior pituitary gland, hypothalamus, or testes. Scratches and inflammation at the base of the penis may indicate lice. Check for nits on the pubic hair.

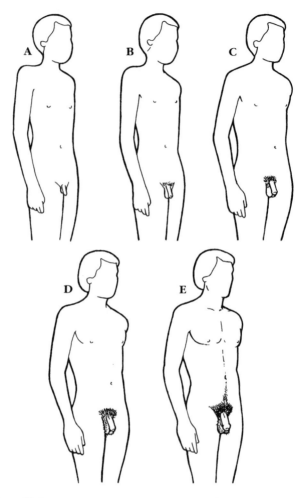

Figure 19-5
Tanner stages in development of male genitalia. **A,** Pre-pubescent. Genitals are the same as those in childhood. **B,** Scrotum and testes enlarge. Scrotal skin reddens. Downy, straight hair grows at base of penis. **C,** Penis, scrotum, and testes enlarge. Hair becomes curly, coarser. **D,** Penis enlarges further. Scrotum darkens. Hair similar to that of an adult but covers smaller area. **E,** Genitals and hair are adultlike.

Related Nursing Diagnoses

Impaired comfort: Related to menses; infection.

Impaired verbal communication: Related to fear; modesty; body changes; knowledge deficit.

Compromised family coping: Related to family history of sexual abuse; adolescent pregnancy; conflict regarding sexual activity.

Interrupted family processes: Related to sexual maturation.

Fear: Related to knowledge deficit; pregnancy; crisis; infection.

Infection: Related to increased sexual contact; multiple sexual partners.

Deficient knowledge: Related to normal development; safe sexual practices; breast self-examination; home contraceptive practices; pregnancy; testicular self-examination.

Self-care deficit: Related to hygiene in uncircumcised boys; hygiene during menses.

Situational low self-esteem: Related to disturbances in body image, self-esteem, role performance, personal identity related to sexual changes.

Ineffective sexuality patterns: Related to sexual maturation; emerging sexual identity.

Impaired skin integrity: Related to infection; discharge; abuse.

Musculoskeletal System

20

The nurse can obtain a great deal of data about the musculoskeletal system by watching the child walk, sit, and carry on various activities during other portions of the health assessment. Specific assessments aid in screening for childhood disorders such as clubfoot, congenital hip dislocation, and scoliosis.

Rationale

Movement is so much a part of a child's activities that it is important to screen for disorders that may affect a child's socialization, exercise patterns, and ability to engage in self-care. Early diagnosis and intervention in disorders such as congenital hip dislocation can possibly prevent more exhaustive treatment as the child grows older.

Anatomy and Physiology

The musculoskeletal system provides support for the body and enables movement. The musculoskeletal system is composed of bones, muscles, tendons, ligaments, cartilage, and joints.

The skeleton arises from mesoderm. At birth the epiphyses of most bones are made of hyaline cartilage. Shortly after birth, secondary ossification centers appear in the epiphyses. The epiphyses ossify, except for the epiphyseal plate, which separates the epiphyses and the diaphyses. The epiphyseal plate is replaced by bone until only the epiphyseal line remains. When the epiphyses are completely ossified, no further bone lengthening occurs.

Muscle fibers are developed by the fourth or fifth month of gestation. The number of muscle fibers remains constant throughout life. Muscle growth is accomplished by increase in the size of the fibers. Muscle mass decreases from one fourth of total body weight at birth to one sixth of total body weight at adolescence.

Transient increases in nonlean mass (subcutaneous fat) occur just before the growth spurt, especially in boys, accompanied by decreases 1 to 2 years later. Lean body mass increases, chiefly muscle, occur after the growth spurt, with the increase greater in males than in females.

Preparation

Inquire whether the infant sustained trauma or injury at birth. Inquire whether there is a family history of bone or joint disorders and whether the child has experienced delays in gross or fine motor development, trauma, joint stiffness and swelling, fever, or pain. If the child has or has had pain, it is important to determine the location, type, intensity, and time of occurrence of the pain. Sharp pain that lessens during rest may indicate injury. Constant dull pain that awakens the child might indicate tumor or infection. Inquire about participation in sports activities (type of sport; level of training involved) and diet.

Minimal clothing assists with assessment of the spine.

Assessment of Musculoskeletal System

Assessment	Findings
If the child is able to walk, observe the gait. Note the presence of casts and braces.	Infants and toddlers tend to walk bowlegged. A wide-based gait is normal in the infant and toddler.
	Clinical Alert
	Limping may indicate congenital dislocation of one hip (especially in toddlers). If both hips are involved, the child has a waddling gait. (Table 20-1 on page 237 lists further indications of congenital hip dislocation.)
	Limping also indicates scoliosis, Legg-Calvé-Perthes disease, infection of the joints of the lower extremities, a slipped capital femoral epiphyses, or stress fractures of the metatarsals.

Assessment	Findings
	Weight bearing on the toes *(pes equinus)* and short heel cords indicate muscular disease or cerebral palsy.
Observe the curve of the infant's or child's spine and note the symmetry of the hips and shoulders. Test for scoliosis by having the child bend forward at the waist and observing the child from front, back, and side.	The spine is normally rounded in the infant younger than 3 months. A lumbar curve forms at 12 to 18 months.
	Lumbar lordosis is normal in young children.
	Clinical Alert
	Kyphosis (hunchback) may indicate wedge-shaped or collapsed vertebrae secondary to myelomeningocele, spinal tumors, Scheuermann's disease, tuberculosis of the spine, or sickle cell anemia. Kyphosis may also indicate habitual slouching.
	The persistence of lateral curvature of the spine indicates scoliosis. If the child can voluntarily correct the curve or if it disappears when the child is recumbent, the curve may be functional. A persistent curve, accompanied by unequal height of the shoulders and iliac crests when the child is standing erect and asymmetric elevation of the scapula when the child is leaning forward (Figure 20-1) indicate structural scoliosis.
Observe the lumbosacral area for abnormalities of the overlying skin (pigmented skin, hairy patches, or dimpling).	Pigmented skin, hairy patches, or dimpling in the lumbosacral area may indicate spina bifida occulta.

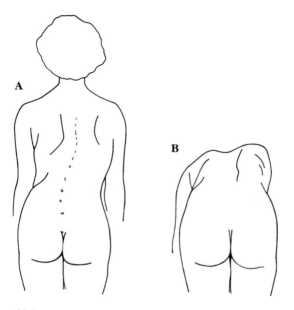

Figure 20-1
Scoliosis. **A,** When child stands, spine assumes lateral curvature and thoracic convexity is present. **B,** When child bends, chest wall on side of convexity is prominent and scapula on side of convexity is elevated.

Assessment	Findings
Note the mobility of the spine, especially the cervical spine.	No resistance or pain should be felt when the child bends or when the neck is flexed or moved from side to side. **Clinical Alert** Pain, crying, or resistance when the neck is flexed indicates meningeal irritation and is known as Brudzinski's sign. Lateral inclination of the head may indicate congenital torticollis.

Assessment	Findings
	Limitations in movement of the cervical spine may indicate cervical fusion, which is found in some children with fetal alcohol syndrome.
	Limitations in shoulder movement and pain across the upper back may be related to packing heavy book bags.
Inspect and palpate the upper extremities. Note the size, color, temperature, range of motion, and mobility of the joints and abnormalities in the upper extremities. Inspect the palmar creases (Figure 20-2).	**Clinical Alert**
	Short, broad extremities, hyperextensible joints, and simian creases may indicate the presence of Down syndrome.
	The Sydney line is found in children with rubella syndrome.
	Abnormal palmar creases may indicate fetal alcohol syndrome.
	Polydactyly (external digits) and syndactyly (webbing) are abnormal findings and may or may not indicate more serious underlying conditions.
	Warmth and tenderness of the joints may indicate rheumatoid arthritis. Tenderness also indicates Lyme disease or Henoch-Schönlein purpura.
	Widening of the wrist joints may indicate rickets.
	Limitation of elbow extension and pain may indicate subluxation of the head of the radius.
Assess the strength of the upper extremities by asking the child to squeeze your crossed fingers.	The strength of the upper extremities should be equal.
	Clinical Alert
	Unilateral weakness may indicate hemiparesis or pain.

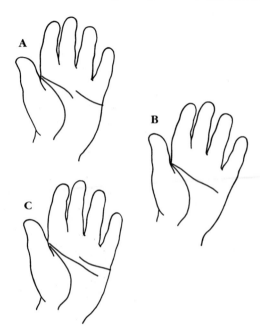

Figure 20-2
Palmar creases. **A,** Normal creases. **B,** Simian crease.
C, Sydney line.

Assessment	Findings
Inspect and palpate the lower extremities. Assess for abnormalities of mobility, length, shape, and pulses.	The feet of infants and toddlers are flat, and the legs are bowed until walking has been firmly established. **Clinical Alert** Fibrosis and contracture of the gluteal and quadriceps muscles occur as complications of intramuscular injections. Observe for limited knee flexion (quadriceps involvement) or hip flexion (gluteal involvement).

Assessment	Findings
Assess for *genu varum* (bowleg) or *genu valgum* (knock-knee) by instructing the child to stand with ankles together.	Knock-knee is present until the child is past 7 years of age. **Clinical Alert** In the child older than 2 years of age, a space greater than 5 cm (2 in) between the knees indicates *genu varum.* A space greater than 7.5 cm (3 in) between the knees in the child older than 7 years indicates *genu valgum.*
Assess for the presence of club-foot by lightly scratching the inner and outer soles of the feet. Observe whether the foot assumes a normal angle (i.e., right angle) to the leg when stimulated.	**Clinical Alert** Return of the foot, after stimulation, to a right angle in relation to the leg may indicate metatarsus varus in an infant with adduction and inversion of the forefoot. Inability of the foot to right itself after stimulation may indicate talipes equinovarus (inversion of the forefoot, plantar flexion, and heel inversion) or talipes calcaneovalgus (eversion of the forefoot and dorsal flexion).
Assess the child for meningeal irritation by flexing the child's hips and then straightening each of the knees (Kernig's sign).	**Clinical Alert** Pain and resistance to straightening of the knees indicates meningeal irritation.
Assess for congenital hip dislocation (see Table 20-1).	
Assess for strength in the lower limbs by asking the child to push against your hands with the soles of the forefeet.	Strength should be symmetric in the lower limbs. **Clinical Alert** Unequal strength may indicate hemiparesis or pain.
Palpate knees for tenderness, warmth, and consistency.	**Clinical Alert** Tenderness, warmth, and boggy consistency may indicate synovitis.

Table 20-1 Assessment for Presence of Congenital Hip Dislocation

Test/Sign	Assessment	Abnormal Findings
Galeazzi or Allis' sign	Place the infant supine with the hips and knees flexed.	The knees are unequal in height. (Finding may not be apparent in the infant younger than 6 weeks.)
Unequal thigh folds	Place the infant or child prone. Observe symmetry of the thigh folds.	Unequal thigh folds.
Ortolani's sign	Place the infant supine. With your thumbs on the inside of both thighs and your fingertips resting over the trochanter muscles, flex both hips and knees. Abduct each knee until the lateral aspects of the knees touch the examining table. This test is reliable in the neonate and may be performed until the child is 1 year of age. It is less reliable in the older infant.	A click or clunk is heard on abduction.
Barlow's test	Place the infant supine. Flex and slightly adduct both hips while lifting the femur and applying pressure to the trochanter. This test is reliable in the neonate.	Instability of hip joints.
Trendelenburg gait	Observe the gait of the child.	When the child bears weight on the affected side, the unaffected side of the pelvis drops (Figure 20-3).

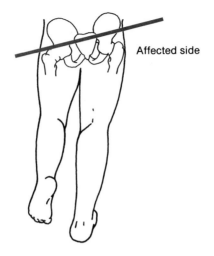

Figure 20-3
Trendelenburg gait.

Assessment	Findings
	Pain, diffuse swelling, and limitation of movement may indicate sprain.
If large amounts of fluid are suspected in the knee, instruct the child or adolescent to lie down. Grasp the patella firmly on each side with the left thumb and index finger. With right fingers, push down on the patella. Feel for a click or fluid wave (ballottement test).	Normal finding is absence of movement of patella. **Clinical Alert** Click or fluid wave indicates large amount of knee joint effusion.
If child or adolescent states knee "locks" or "gives way," perform McMurray's test. With the child supine, ask the child to flex the affected knee and hip. Place	Absence of pain and clicking are normal findings. **Clinical Alert** Clicking or pain may indicate a torn meniscus of the knee joint.

Assessment	Findings
the thumb and index finger of one hand on either side of the knee; with the other hand, rotate the lower leg and foot laterally, holding the heel. Slowly extend the knee, noting pain or clicking. Rotate the lower leg and foot medially, observing for pain and clicking.	

Related Nursing Diagnoses

Anxiety: Related to pain secondary to injury; surgery; disease.

Impaired comfort: Pain related to injury; surgery; disease; position.

Risk for impaired skin integrity: Related to immobility, casts.

Deficient knowledge: Related to care of the child with braces or casts.

Impaired physical mobility: Secondary to surgery; injury; disease; corrective devices.

Impaired parenting: Related to skill deficit; stress.

Self-care deficit: Feeding, bathing/hygiene, dressing secondary to pain; immobility; weakness; corrective devices.

Self-esteem: Disturbance in body image, role performance related to limitations in mobility; physical disability.

Impaired walking: Related to acute or chronic illness; surgery; disability.

Nervous System

21

Assessment of the nervous system involves observation and testing of mental status, motor functioning, sensory functioning, cranial nerve functioning, reflexes, and infant automatisms. The thoroughness of assessment depends on the presenting complaint, contributing data from the health assessment, the reason for the assessment, the condition, and the child's age.

Much of the neurologic assessment can be integrated with other areas of the assessment. Parents can be valuable aides in performing the neurologic assessment of a child because they are more aware of the child's usual functioning. Parental concerns are important in alerting health professionals to delays, impairments, and need for anticipatory guidance.

In performing the neurologic assessment, the nurse must be aware of age-appropriate levels of functioning.

Rationale

A thorough neurologic assessment is necessary whenever a child has sustained a fall or has suffered an injury to the head or spine, or complains of headaches or has a temperature of unknown origin. Children who have an apparent developmental delay or impairment and those with identified neurologic disorders should also undergo neurologic assessment. Neurologic impairment can delay a child's development and functioning and must be identified early to minimize long-term disability.

Anatomy and Physiology

The nervous system is a complex integrated system, and its scope is beyond that of this text. Essentially the nervous system is composed of the brain, spinal cord, and peripheral nervous system. The brain is divided into the brainstem, the cerebrum, and the cerebellum. Except for the first cranial nerve, the cranial nerves emerge from the brainstem. The brainstem and the spinal cord are continuous. Consciousness arises from interaction between the cerebrum and brainstem. The cerebellum is primarily responsible for coordination. The full number of adult nerve cells is established midway through the prenatal period. Neurons, responsible for memory, consciousness, sensory and motor responses, and thought control, increase in size but not number after birth. Glial cells increase in both size and number until the age of 4 years. Dendrites, responsible for the transmission of impulses across synapses, increase in number and branchings. Axons increase in length. The size of the brain increases from 325 gm (11 oz) at birth to 1000 gm (2.2 lb) by 1 year of age (the adult brain weighs 1400 gm, or approximately 3 lb). Myelinization, begun in the fourth month of gestation, progresses throughout early infancy and childhood, until the child is able to move voluntarily and to engage in higher cortical functions. The order in which myelinization occurs corresponds to the normal sequence of development.

Equipment for Assessment of Nervous System

Two safety pins
Closed jars containing solutions with distinctive odors
Cotton balls
Reflex hammer

Preparation

Ask whether there is a family history of genetic disorders, learning disorders, or birth defects. Inquire whether the mother had difficulties during pregnancy or delivery. Ask the parent about prenatal history, consumption of drugs (such as alcohol, cocaine, heroin, and marijuana) during pregnancy, type of delivery, birth weight of the infant or child, and whether the infant or child had problems after birth. Ask whether the child has or has had recurrent headaches, seizures, irritability, or hyperactivity. If the child has sustained an injury, determine the time of occurrence, the events surrounding the injury, the area of impact, and whether consciousness was lost.

Assessment of Mental Status

Mental status can be assessed formally and informally throughout the examination and includes intellectual or cognitive functioning, thought and perceptions, mood, appearance, and behavior. Intellectual functioning can be formally assessed through the use of the Denver II test (see Chapter 22), which is administered at specified intervals in some agencies but can be administered any time a problem is suspected. Illness, injury, a strange environment, cultural and language differences, and the examiner's approach can all influence intellectual functioning, mood, and understanding, so the nurse should compare findings against the parent's observations of the child's behavior.

Assessment	Findings
Level of Consciousness (LOC)	Normal children will score 15 on the Glasgow Coma Scale.
Level of consciousness (LOC) remains the most reliable and earliest indicator of changes in neurologic status and is a less variable indicator than vital signs, reflexes, and motor activity. LOC can be assessed using a pediatric version of the Glasgow Coma Scale (Figure 21-1). Responses in each category are rated on a scale from 1 to 5. Whenever possible, have a parent present because a child may not respond actively to an unfamiliar person in an unfamiliar environment. It is also important to ask the parent about the child's normal level of responsiveness.	**Clinical Alert** A score of 8 or less on the Glasgow Coma Scale indicates coma.
Posture and Motor Behavior	
Assess the child's level of activity (pace, range, character	Motor behavior will vary with the age of the child and stage

NEUROLOGIC ASSESSMENT

Pupils	Right	Size		++ = Brisk
		Reaction		+ = Sluggish
	Left	Size		− = No reaction
		Reaction		C = Eye closed by swelling

Pupil scale (mm): 1, 2, 3, 4, 6, 7, 8

	GLASGOW COMA SCALE		
Eyes open	Spontaneously	4	
	To speech	3	
	To pain	2	
	None	1	
Best motor response	Obeys commands	6	
	Localizes pain	5	
	Flexion withdrawal	4	
	Flexion abnormal	3	
	Extension	2	
	None	1	

Usually record best arm or age-appropriate response

Best response to auditory and/or visual stimulus	>2 years		<2 years
	Orientation	5	5 Smiles, listens, follows
	Confused	4	4 Cries, consolable
	Inappropriate words	3	3 Inappropriate persistent cry
	Incomprehensible words	2	2 Agitated, restless
	None	1	1 No response
	Endotracheal tube or trach	T	

COMA SCALE TOTAL

HAND GRIP:
Equal
Unequal
R_____L
Weakness

LOC:
Alert/oriented x4
Sleepy
Irritable
Comatose
Disoriented
Combative
Lethargic
Awake
Sleeping
Drowsy
Agitated

MUSCLE TONE:
Normal
Arching
Spastic
Flaccid
Weak
Decorticate
Decerebrate
Other _____

EYE MOVEMENT:
Normal
Nystagmus
Strabismus
Other _____

FONTANEL/WINDOW:
Soft
Flat
Sunken
Tense
Bulging
Closed
Other _____

MOOD/AFFECT:
Happy
Content
Quiet
Withdrawn
Sad
Flat
Hostile

Figure 21-1
Pediatric adaptation of Glasgow Coma Scale.
(From Wong DL et al: *Whaley & Wong's nursing care of infants and children,* ed 6, St Louis, 1999, Mosby.)

Assessment	Findings
of movements), control of impulses (avoids interrupting and blurting out, waits turn), appropriateness of behavior to situation and developmental stage, repetitive movements (rocking, head banging), presence of culturally appropriate eye contact and interaction, withdrawal, cooperativeness, and argumentativeness.	of development, what is acceptable within the family, and cultural norms. **Clinical Alert** Hyperactivity, irritability, and diminished impulse control may indicate attention deficit disorder or fetal alcohol syndrome. Aggressiveness, irritability, disobedience, and emotional lability may indicate post-traumatic syndrome when injury has occurred. Hyperactivity, hypoactivity, and other behavioral changes can accompany the use of commonly abused drugs (Table 21-1). Withdrawal, diminished eye contact (unless culturally appropriate), slumped shoulders, and slowed movements may indicate depression.
Hygiene and Grooming Observe hygiene and grooming in older children and adolescents. Inquire if there have been changes in grooming habits lately that are of concern.	**Clinical Alert** Neglect of personal hygiene may indicate family stress, depression, or substance abuse.
Mood Observe moods and intensity of moods. If depression is suspected, inquire of parent or child: • What do you do when you get mad? Frustrated? Do you use alcohol/drugs	**Clinical Alert** Persistent sadness, extreme irritability, preoccupation with death, reckless or antisocial behavior, putting affairs in order (giving away possessions), and sudden cheerfulness may indicate increased risk for suicide.

Table 21-1 Behaviors and Terms Associated with Psychoactive Substance Abuse

Substance	Terms Associated with Substance	Behaviors and Physical Responses Associated with Intoxication	Developmental Effects of Prenatal Exposure
Alcohol	Mountain dew, alley juice, moonshine, sauce, booze, hootch	Decreased alertness, slurred speech, nausea, vertigo, staggering, emotional lability, stupor, unconsciousness	Fetal alcohol effects, fetal alcohol syndrome
Barbiturate	Downers, goofers, barbs, idiot pills, nimlue, peanuts, sleepers	Drowsiness, relaxation, slurred speech, slow and shallow respirations, pulse rate and blood pressure lowered, cold and clammy skin, depression, poor judgment, motor impairment	Unknown
Narcotics	Dreamer, dust, hard stuff, morf, white stuff, Big Harry, horse, joy powder, smack, stuff, white lady	Euphoria, clouding of consciousness, dreamlike state, respiratory depression, pupillary construction, cyanosis, needle marks on arms	Increased rate of sudden infant death syndrome (SIDS), hyperactivity
Cocaine	C, candy, cecil, coke, crack, nose, nose candy, rock, snow, stardust, white horse	Euphoria, disinhibition, irritability, anxiety, insomnia, lack of energy and motivation, psychomotor retardation, slow pulse and respirations, dilated pupils, increased blood pressure, hyperactivity, hypersexuality	Developmental delay, increased risk of sudden infant death syndrome, hyperactivity, hypertonia (children under 2 years), head circumference smaller (under 2 years of age)

Continued

Table 21-1 Behaviors and Terms Associated with Psychoactive Substance Abuse—cont'd

Substance	Terms Associated with Substance	Behaviors and Physical Responses Associated with Intoxication	Developmental Effects of Prenatal Exposure
Amphetamines	Beans, berries, black beauties, browns, co-pilots, dice, drives, eye openers, led rollers, pep pills, speed, white crossed, zip	Sweating, dilated pupils, agitation, irritability, insomnia, hyperactivity, paranoia, confusion, aggressiveness, restlessness, anorexia, slurred speech	Poor school performance
Hallucinogens (LSD, PCP, PMT, STP)	Acid, cube, heavenly haze, sugar, angel dust, elephant, goon, magic mist, hog	Vomiting, tremors, panic, agitation, depression, aggression, nystagmus, sweating, paranoia, elevated blood pressure, hallucinations	Unknown
Cannabis	Bush, joint, reefer, pot, smoke, straw, weed, hemp, hooter, jive	Laughter, confusion, panic, drowsiness, reddened eyes, increased vital signs, increased appetite, blurred vision, depression, irritability, emotional swings, decreased motivation, impaired memory	Prenatal exposure: Infants can exhibit symptoms of withdrawal after delivery (irritability, disturbed sleep).
Inhalants		Giddiness, drowsiness, headache, nausea, fainting, loss of consciousness, respiratory arrest, muscular weakness	Unknown
Nicotine		Headache; nausea; increased pulse, blood pressure, and muscle tone	Poor school performance, increased risk of sudden infant death syndrome

Assessment	Findings
sometimes? If so, when do you use drugs/alcohol? Do you miss school sometimes to use drugs/alcohol? Have your friends changed? Have your grades changed?	Social isolation, dropping grades, and shifts in peer group may indicate alcohol/drug abuse or other addictive activities.
What things make you scared? What do you do when you get scared?	Well-described plans, including who will be at the funeral and the funeral plans, may indicate significant risk for suicide.
What kinds of things do you worry about?	
Have you thought about hurting yourself? Others? If so, how would you do it?	
Have you tried to kill yourself before? Did you receive any help afterward?	

Assessment of Motor Function

Motor function can be assessed during assessment of the musculoskeletal system.

Assessment	Findings
Observe the infant or child for obvious abnormalities that may influence motor functioning. Specifically, observe the size and shape of the head and inspect the spine for sacs and tufts of hair.	**Clinical Alert** A large head, enlarged frontal area, and tense fontanels (if open) may indicate hydrocephalus. A dimple with a tuft of hair or a sac protruding from the spinal column may indicate spina bifida occulta. A small head or microcephaly is associated with chromosomal abnormalities, prenatal exposure to toxic agents, maternal infections, and trauma during the perinatal period or infancy.

Assessment	Findings
Test muscle strength and symmetry by asking the child to squeeze your fingers, press soles of feet against your hands, and push away pressure exerted on arms and legs.	**Clinical Alert** Report any asymmetry.
Place all joints through range of motion. Note flaccidity or spasticity.	Infants normally have the most flexible range of motion. All school-aged children should be able to perform these activities. **Clinical Alert** Retroflexion of the head, stiffness of the neck, and extension of the extremities accompanies the meningeal irritation of meningitis and intracranial hemorrhage. Head lag after 4 months is an early sign of neurologic damage. Hypotonia is associated with Down syndrome.
Cerebellar function can be tested by asking the child to hop, skip, or walk heel-to-toe.	**Clinical Alert** Leaning to one side during a Romberg's test indicates cerebellar dysfunction.
A *Romberg's test* can be performed by asking the child to stand still, eyes closed and arms at side. Stand near the child to catch the child if leaning occurs.	

Assessment of Sensory Function

Sensory function is assessed during testing of cranial nerve function.

Assessment of Cranial Nerve Function

The function of most of the cranial nerves can be evaluated during other areas of the health assessment (Table 21-2). Particular attention is paid to function of the cranial nerves when neurologic impairment is possible, suspected, or actually present, and should be a routine part of assessment in a child with a head injury.

Assessment of the cranial nerves varies with the child's developmental and cognitive levels. Testing of several functions depends on the child's ability to understand and cooperate; therefore, such functions cannot be tested in the infant or young child.

Assessment of Deep Tendon Reflexes

Assessment of deep tendon reflexes (Table 21-3) provides information about the intactness of the reflex area. Compare the symmetry and strength of reflexes. Superficial reflexes such as the abdominal reflex, anal reflex, and cremasteric reflex can also be evaluated (Table 21-3), but are usually assessed during other areas of the health assessment. Findings from assessment of deep tendon and superficial reflexes are variable in infancy. Their absence or intensity is not diagnostically significant unless asymmetry is present.

Assessment of Infant Reflexes

Infant reflexes or automatisms (Table 21-4) are particularly useful in assessing the function of the central nervous system. Reflexes should be formally assessed if there is any suggestion of a central nervous disorder. Many reflexes can be assessed during other parts of the health assessment. Knowledge of the reflex aids in education of the parents.

Assessment of Pain

The response of children to pain follows developmental patterns (Table 21-5) and is influenced by temperament, coping abilities, and previous exposure to pain and painful procedures. When assessing pain, the use of various assessment strategies aids in obtaining a more accurate assessment of the pain. These strategies

Text continued on p. 260

Table 21-2 Testing of Cranial Nerve Function

Cranial Nerve	Assessment of Function	Area of Health Assessment into Which Testing Can Be Integrated
I Olfactory	Have the child close eyes and, blocking one nostril at a time, correctly identify distinctive odors (e.g., coffee, oranges).	Head and neck
II Optic*	Check the child's visual acuity, perception of light and color, and peripheral vision. Examine the optic disk.	Eye
III Oculomotor*	Check pupil size and reactivity. Inspect the eyelid for position when open. Have the child follow light or a bright toy through the six cardinal positions of gaze.	Eye
IV Trochlear†	Have the child move eyes downward and inward.	Eye
V Trigeminal*	Palpate the temple and jaw as the child bites down. Assess for symmetry and strength. Determine if the child can detect light touch over the cheeks (a young infant roots when the cheek areas near the mouth are touched). Approaching from the side, touch the colored portion of the eye lightly with a wisp of cotton to test the blink and corneal reflexes.	Eye
VI Abducens†	Ask the child to look sideways. Assess the ability to move eyes laterally.	Eye

Cranial Nerve	Assessment	Location
VII Facial*	Test the child's ability to identify sweet (sugar), sour (lemon juice), or bitter (quinine) solutions with the anterior tongue. Assess motor function by asking the older child to smile, puff out the cheeks, or show the teeth. (Observe the infant while smiling and crying.)	Head and neck
VIII Acoustic	Test the child's hearing (see Chapter 12).	Ear
IX Glossopharyngeal†	Test the child's ability to identify the taste of solutions on the posterior tongue.	Head and neck
X Vagus	Assess the child for hoarseness and ability to swallow. Touch a tongue blade to the posterior pharynx to determine if the gag reflex is present (cranial nerves IX and X both participate in this response). *Do not stimulate the gag reflex if there is any suspicion of epiglottitis.* Check that the uvula is in the midline.	Head and neck
XI Accessory†	Have the child attempt to turn the head to the side against resistance. Ask the child to shrug shoulders while downward pressure is applied.	Head and neck
XII Hypoglossal†	Ask the child to stick out the tongue. Inspect the tongue for midline deviation. (Observe the infant's tongue for lateral deviation when crying and laughing.) Listen for the child's ability to pronounce "r" (rabbit, run, Robert). Place a tongue blade against the side of child's tongue and ask the child to move it away. Assess for strength.	Head and neck

*Some portions of function can be assessed in infants and in younger children.
†Only older children can participate in testing.

Table 21-3   Assessment of Deep and Superficial Reflexes

Reflex	Method of Assessment	Usual Finding
Deep Tendon Reflexes		
Biceps	Partially flex the child's forearm. Place your thumb over the antecubital space and strike with the reflex hammer (Figure 21-2, *A*).	Forearm flexes slightly.
Triceps	Bend the child's arm at the elbow while supporting the forearm. Strike the triceps tendon above the elbow (Figure 21-2, *B*).	Forearm extends slightly.
Brachioradialis	Place the child's arm and hand in a relaxed position with the palm down. Strike the radius 2.5 cm (1 inch) above the wrist.	Forearm flexes and palm turns upward.
Knee jerk or patellar	Have the child sit on a table or on the parent's lap with legs flexed and dangling. Strike the patellar tendon just below the kneecap.	Lower leg extends.

Achilles	Have the child sit on a table or on the parent's lap with legs flexed and support the foot lightly. Strike the Achilles tendon.	Foot plantar flexes (points downward). Rapid, rhythmic plantar flexion of the foot may occur in newborn infants (up to 10 flexions may be noted).
Superficial Reflexes		
Abdominal	Stroke the skin toward the umbilicus. Assess the reflex in all four quadrants. The abdominal reflex may not be present for the first 6 months. (Can be incorporated into assessment of the abdomen.)	Umbilicus moves toward the stimulus.
Cremasteric	Stroke the upper inner thigh. (Can be integrated into assessment of the abdominal or genital area.)	Testes retract into the inguinal canal.
Anal	Stimulate the skin in the perianal area. (Can be incorporated into assessment of the rectal area.)	Brisk contraction of the anal sphincter occurs.

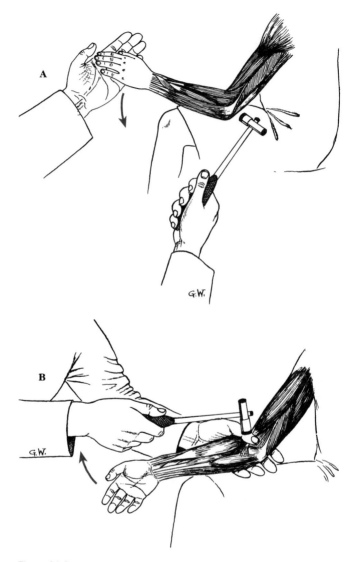

Figure 21-2
Assessment of deep tendon reflexes. A, Triceps. **B,** Biceps.
(From Whaley LF, Wong DL: *Nursing care of infants and children,* ed 4, St Louis, 1991, Mosby.)

Table 21-4   Infant Reflexes (Automatisms)

Reflex	Description	Method of Assessment	Significance of Findings
Blinking (dazzle)	Closes eyelids in response to bright light. Present during first year of life.	Shine light into infant's eyes.	Absence of reflex suggests blindness.
Babinski's sign	Toes fan and big toe dorsiflexes. Present until 2 years of age.	Stroke sole of foot along outer edge, beginning from heel.	Fanning of toes and dorsiflexion of great toe after 2 years of age suggests lesion in extrapyramidal tract.
Crawling	Infant makes crawling movements with arms and legs when placed on abdomen.	Place infant prone on flat surface.	Asymmetry of movements suggests neurologic disorder.
Dance or stepping	Infant's feet move up and down when feet lightly touch firm surface. Present for first 4-8 weeks.	Hold infant so that feet lightly touch firm surface.	Persistence of reflex beyond 4-8 weeks is abnormal.
Extrusion	Tongue extends outward when touched. Present until 4 months of age.	Touch tongue with tip of tongue blade.	Persistent extension of tongue may indicate Down syndrome.

Continued

Table 21-4 Infant Reflexes (Automatisms)—cont'd

Reflex	Description	Method of Assessment	Significance of Findings
Galant's (trunk incurvation)	Back moves toward side that is stimulated. Present for first 4-8 weeks.	Stroke infant's back along side of spine from shoulder to buttocks.	Absence of reflex may indicate transverse spinal cord lesions.
Moro's	Arms extend, fingers fan, head is thrown back, and legs may flex weakly. Arms return to center with hands clasped. Spine and lower extremities extend. Strongest during first 2 months. Disappears at 3-4 months.	Change infant's position abruptly or jar table.	Persistence of reflex beyond 4 months suggests brain damage. Persistence beyond 6 months highly indicates brain damage. Asymmetry of responses indicates hemiparesis, fracture of clavicle, or injury to brachial plexus. Absence of response in lower extremities indicates congenital hip dislocation or low spinal cord injury.
Neck righting	When infant is supine, shoulder and trunk and then pelvis turn toward direction in which infant is turned. Persists for first 10 months.	Place infant supine. Attempt to attract infant's attention to one side.	Absence or persistence beyond 10 months suggests central nervous system disorders.

Reflex			
Palmar grasp	Infant's fingers curve around finger placed in infant's palm from ulnar side. Palmar grasp disappears by 3-4 months.	Place finger into infant's palm from ulnar side. If reflex is weak or absent, offer infant bottle or soother because sucking enhances reflex.	Asymmetric flexion indicates paralysis. Persistence of grasp reflex indicates cerebral disorder.
Rooting	Infant turns in direction that cheek is stroked. Reflex disappears at 3-4 months, but may persist for up to 12 months, especially during sleep.	Stroke corners of infant's mouth or midline of lips	Absence of reflex indicates severe neurologic disorder. Exaggerated rooting reflex together with ineffective sucking is associated with cocaine-dependent mothers.
Startle	Infant extends and flexes arms in response to loud noise. Hands remain clenched. Reflex disappears after 4 months of age unless there are neurologic impairments. Infants with neurologic impairments may evidence increased sensitivity to sound.	Claps hands loudly.	Absence of reflex indicates hearing impairment.

Continued

Table 21-4   Infant Reflexes (Automatisms)—cont'd

Reflex	Description	Method of Assessment	Significance of Findings
Sucking	Infant sucks strongly in response to stimulation. Reflex persists during infancy and may occur during sleep without stimulation.	Offer infant bottle or soother.	Weak or absent reflex suggests developmental delay or neurologic abnormality.
Tonic neck	Infant assumes fencing position when head is turned to one side. Arm and leg extend on side to which head is turned and flex on opposite side. Normally reflex should not occur each time head is turned. Appears at approximately 2 months, disappears at 6 months.	Turn head quickly to one side.	It is considered abnormal if response occurs each time head is turned. Persistence indicates major cerebral damage.

Table 21-5 Developmental Responses to Pain

Age	Motor Response	Expressive Response	Ability to Anticipate Pain
Young infants	Generalized. Includes thrashing, rigidity, exaggerated reflex withdrawal, lack of sucking, disorganized sucking, starts to eat or drink and discontinues.	Cries loudly, closes eyes tightly, opens mouth in squarish manner, grimaces.	No link between approaching stimulus and pain.
Older infants	Localized. Withdrawal of affected area. Sucking and feeding behaviors as for young infants.	As for young infant except eyes may be open.	Physical resistance after painful stimulus occurs.
Young children	Thrashes arms, legs. Uncooperative, reluctant to move, lies rigid, guards area, restless.	Cries, screams loudly, moans, verbalizes pain, clings to support person, asks for support, irritable.	Anticipates pain.
School-age	Includes behaviors found in young child as well as muscular rigidity (clenched fists, body stiffness, closed eyes, frowning), muscle tension, and withdrawal.	Includes responses found in young child as well as stalling or bargaining behavior.	Behaviors seen less before procedure; more pronounced during pain experience.
Adolescents	Less motor activity than younger child. Demonstrates muscle tension, body control.	Uses more sophisticated language to verbalize pain. Less verbal protest.	Uses anticipation to prepare self.

include questioning the child (in words that are appropriate to developmental level and language) and the parents, observing behavioral and physiologic responses, using pain scales (Table 21-6). PEPPS (Table 21-7) is a pain measurement tool that is useful with toddlers and for taking and evaluating action. Headache is a common symptom in children and may indicate several disorders (Table 21-8).

Related Nursing Diagnoses

Constipation: Related to spinal cord lesions; neurologic disease.

Impaired comfort: Pain secondary to increased intracranial pressure.

Impaired verbal communication: Secondary to deafness; neurologic impairment.

Compromised family coping: Compromised related to situational crisis; temporary family disorganization.

Diversional deficit: Related to decreased mobility; difficulty in coordinating movements; physical weakness.

Interrupted family processes: Related to situational crisis.

Delayed growth and development: Related to diversional deficit; cerebral impairment.

Risk for injury: Related to impaired coordination; immobility.

Impaired physical mobility: Secondary to neurologic injury; congenital defects.

Impaired parenting: Related to skill deficit; knowledge deficit; family stress.

Disturbed sleep pattern: Related to pain; depression; drug use.

Risk for self-directed violence: Related to impulsivity; depression; situational crisis; disturbed thought processes.

Risk for other-directed violence: Related to impulsivity; compromised coping strategies; situational crisis; disturbed thought processes.

Self-care deficit: Feeding, bathing/hygiene, dressing/grooming, toileting related to muscle weakness; immobility; developmental lag.

Low self-esteem: Related to disturbance in body image, physical limitations; developmental delay; perception of disabilities.

Impaired skin integrity: Actual or high risk for complication related to immobility; urinary incontinence; fecal incontinence.

Social isolation: Related to impaired mobility; disturbance in self-concept; depression.

Altered thought processes: Secondary to cerebral dysfunction; drugs; mental health issues.

Impaired urinary elimination: Related to ineffective urinary sphincter muscle.

Table 21-6 Pain Assessment Tools for Children and Adolescents

Tool	Instructions
Adolescent pediatric pain tool (APPT)	Ask adolescent to color in areas of pain on anterior and posterior body outlines. Ask adolescent to make marks as big or small as pain.
Wong-Baker FACES pain rating scale	

0	1	2	3	4	5
No Hurt	Hurts little bit	Hurts little more	Hurts even more	Hurts whole lot	Hurts worst

Explain to the child that each face is for a person who feels happy because he has no pain (hurt) or sad because he has some or a lot of pain. Face 0 is very happy because he doesn't hurt at all. Face 1 hurts just a little bit. Face 2 hurts a little more. Face 3 hurts even more. Face 4 hurts a whole lot. Face 5 hurts as much as you can imagine, although you don't have to be crying to feel this bad. Ask the child to choose the face that best describes how he or she is feeling.

Recommended for children age 3 years and older.

| Numeric scale | Ask the child to rate pain on a line from 0 to 10, with 0 being no hurt and 10 being the worst possible pain. Useful for children who know how to count and know what is more or less. |

From Murphy E et al: Development of a pain assessment scale for the preverbal, early verbal child. Abstract no. 160; presented at the Third International Symposium on Pediatric Pain, Children and Pain: Integrating Science and Care, Philadelphia, June 1994, copyright © WB Saunders Co. FACES from Wong DL et al: *Whaley & Wong's nursing care of infants and children*, ed 6, St Louis, 1999, Mosby.

Table 21-7 Preverbal, Early Verbal Pediatric Pain Scale

Heart Rate

4—>40 beats/min above baseline
3—31-40 beats above baseline
2—21-30 beats above baseline
1—10-20 beats above baseline
0—baseline range

Facial

4—Severe grimace; brows lowered, tightly drawn together; eyes tightly closed
2—Grimace; brows drawn together, eyes partially closed, squinting
0—Relaxed facial expression

Cry (Audible/Visible)

4—Screaming
3—Sustained crying
2—Intermittent crying
1—Whimpering, groaning, fussiness
0—No cry

Consolability/State of Restfulness

4—Unable to console, restlessness, sustained movement
2—Able to console, distract with difficulty, intermittent restlessness, irritability
1—Distractable, easy to console, intermittent fussiness
0—Pleasant, well integrated

Body Posture

4—Sustained arching, flailing, thrashing and/or kicking
3—Intermittent or sustained movement with or without periods of rigidity
2—Localization with extension or flexion or stiff and nonmoving
1—Clenched fists, curled toes and/or reaching for, touching wound or area
0—Body at rest, relaxed positioning

Sociability

4—Absent eye contact, response to voice and/or touch
2—With effort, responds to voice and/or touch, makes eye contact, difficult to obtain and maintain
0—Responds to voice and/or touch, makes eye contact and/or smiles, easy to obtain and maintain; sleeping

Sucking/Feeding

2—Lack of sucking, refusing food, fluids
1—Disorganized sucking, attempting to eat or drink but discontinues
0—Sucking, drinking and/or eating well
0—N/A; NPO and/or does not use oral stimuli

Total score: _____

From Murphy E et al: Development of a pain assessment scale for the preverbal, early verbal child. Abstract No. 160. Presented at the Third International Symposium on Pediatric Pain, Children and Pain: Integrating Science and Care, Philadelphia, June 1994, copyright © WB Saunders Co.

Table 21-8   Characteristics and Etiologies of Headaches in Childhood and Adolescence

Characteristics of Pain	Location	Factors that Aggravate or Provoke	Associated Symptoms	Possible Etiology
Aching, mild, diffuse, tightness and pressure; gradual onset	Usually bilateral; may be generalized; may involve back of head and neck	• School and relationship stressors • Long periods in one position (e.g., working at a computer; playing video games)	• Depression • Anxiety	Tension headache
Aching, progressive, recurrent; worse on arising	Occipital or frontal areas	• Lowering head • Bowel movements, coughing, sneezing	• Vomiting, with or without feeding • Decreased appetite • Increasingly projectile vomiting • Clumsiness • Changes in reflexia • Spasticity • Irritability • Seizures • Weakness • Positive Babinski sign	Brain tumor

Aching, throbbing, variable severity, may be recurrent	Above eye (frontal sinus); in cheek-bones, over gums (maxillary sinus)	• Bending • Coughing • Sneezing • Jarring the head	• Fever • Nasal discharge • Nasal congestion • Halitosis	Sinusitus
Aching, steady, dull, in and around eyes	Around and over eyes	• Activities requiring use of eyes such as reading, schoolwork, video games, television	• Child may say eyes are tired • Redness of conjunctiva • Frequent rubbing of eyes • Squinting • Clumsiness • Nausea following close work	Errors of refraction; strabismus
Steady, severe; abrupt onset, often after falling asleep; clustered over days or a week, with relief for weeks or months	One sided; high along the nose; over and behind the eye	• May be provoked by alcohol use	• Closes one eye • Coryza • Reddening and tearing of the eye	Cluster headaches

Continued

Table 21-8 Characteristics and Etiologies of Headaches in Childhood and Adolescence—cont'd

Characteristics of Pain	Location	Factors that Aggravate or Provoke	Associated Symptoms	Possible Etiology
Steady, aching; gradual onset following injury to head; more common in infancy than in older children	Variable location	• Injury, sometimes forgotten because of passage of time	• Alterations in levels of consciousness • Irritability • Difficulty feeding • Excessive crying • Weakness along one side	Subdural hematoma
Severe, worsening, interferes with sleep	Variable	• Injury to the head, often to the parietotemporal region	• Possible loss of consciousness at time of injury • Drowsiness; difficult to arouse • Confusion • Difficulty with speaking • Irritability, crying • Unsteady gait (older child) • Refusal of feeding • Nausea	Epidural hemorrhage

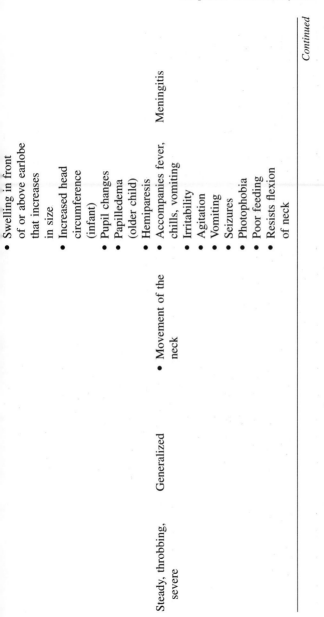

| Steady, throbbing, severe | Generalized | • Movement of the neck | • Swelling in front of or above earlobe that increases in size
• Increased head circumference (infant)
• Pupil changes
• Papilledema (older child)
• Hemiparesis
• Accompanies fever, chills, vomiting
• Irritability
• Agitation
• Vomiting
• Seizures
• Photophobia
• Poor feeding
• Resists flexion of neck | Meningitis |

Continued

Table 21-8   Characteristics and Etiologies of Headaches in Childhood and Adolescence—cont'd

Characteristics of Pain	Location	Factors that Aggravate or Provoke	Associated Symptoms	Possible Etiology
			• Positive Kernig's and Brudzinski's signs	
Throbbing, aching, variable severity, rapid onset	Usually frontal or temporal, but may be occipital; may start behind eye and radiate outward; may be one or both sides	• Alcohol • Some foods (chocolate milk, cheese, soft drinks, food additives) • Tension • Premenstrual • Noise, bright lights	• Nausea, vomiting • Abdominal pain • Visual disturbances • Local weakness • Sensory disturbances	Migraine
Variable quality and severity; post head injury	May be localized	• Mental and physical activity • Excitement • Bending • Alcohol • Noise, lights	• Can occur following injury to the head • Poor concentration • Irritability • Restlessness • Fatigue	Post concussion

GENERAL ASSESSMENT

IV

Development

22

Development is multifactorial and is the interplay among temperament, environment, and biophysical factors. Many observations about development can be made informally during the health interview and during the neurologic and musculoskeletal assessments; however, some observations need to be made more formally using tools such as the Denver II and other objective tests.

The nurse needs to be aware that *"normal" encompasses a wide range of behavior at any given stage* and that delays in development can rarely be attributed to only one factor. Knowledge of behaviors that can be expected at various stages is essential to assessment of development.

Rationale

Complete periodic, systematic assessment of development enables early detection of problems, identification of parental and child concerns, anticipatory guidance, and teaching about age-appropriate expected behaviors. Judgments about an infant's or child's development must *never* rest solely on one assessment of development. Illness, stress, the examiner's approach, and a strange environment can alter a child's usual performance.

Preparation

Ask the parent to describe the infant's or child's development. Inquire whether the parent has specific concerns about the infant's or child's development. Ask about the mother's prenatal history, including miscarriages, stillbirths, exposure to medications or radiation, drug or alcohol use, maternal endocrine disorders, toxemia, hydramnios, infection, or abnormal bleeding. Inquire about the birth history of the infant or child, including type of delivery, fetal distress, birth weight, prematurity, respiratory problems, jaundice, hypoglycemia, seizures, irritability, poor muscle tone, or feeding problems. Inquire about family history of health concerns.

Assessment of Development Using the Denver II Screening Test

The Denver II is not an IQ test, but a series of standard developmental tasks that are used for children from birth to 6 years to determine how a child compares developmentally with other children of the same age. The test assesses personal, social, fine motor, adaptive, language, and gross motor skills and is useful for monitoring children who are at risk for developmental delays. The tests do not tell *why* developmental delays have occurred.

Equipment for Assessment with Denver Screening Tests

Approved Denver II manuals, test kit, and forms.

Method of Assessment

1. Draw a line from top to bottom of the Denver II test form (Appendix A) in the appropriate age slot.
2. Test all items intersected by the vertical or age line. If a number appears on an item, refer to the back of the sheet for specific instructions.
3. Score each item that is administered as pass, fail, refusal, or no opportunity.
4. Score the behavior rating scale.

Significance of Findings

All children are not expected to pass all items. If a child fails one or more items that fall completely to the left of the age line, consider the child's developmental history and health history before deciding whether to retest at a later date.

Assessment of Growth and Development

Assessment of development requires knowledge of what can be expected at various stages in development. Table 22-1 gives a general summary of normal growth and development that can be used during observation of an infant or child.

Related Nursing Diagnoses

Anxiety: Related to separation from parents; peer relationships; achievement; sexual development; independence; parenting.

Ineffective coping: Related to poor self-esteem; developmental tasks; physical and emotional changes; increasing independence from family; peer relationships; heterosexual relationships; sexual awareness; career choices; leaving home.

Compromised family coping: Related to lack of knowledge about normal child development; adolescent rebellion.

Delayed growth and development: Related to physical or cognitive disability; lack of stimulation; illness; inadequate nutrition; abuse or neglect.

Grieving: Related to changes in life-style; child leaving home; loss of image of infant as healthy.

Risk for injury: Related to home environmental hazards; use of bicycles, automobiles; use of drugs, alcohol; increasing independence in activities.

Deficient knowledge: Related to growth and development of the infant or child; contraception.

Parental role conflict: Related to needs precipitated by growth and development of the child or adolescent.

Risk for impaired parenting: Related to lack of knowledge about growth and development; difficulty adjusting parenting to developmental needs of child or adolescent.

Altered sexuality patterns: Related to the physical and emotional changes of adolescence.

Table 22-1   Summary of Normal Growth and Development

Age	Physical/Motor	Language	Cognition	Socialization
1 month	Average weekly weight gain 140-200 gm (5-6 oz) until 6 months of age. Average monthly gain in length 2.5 cm (1 in) until 6 months of age. Obligate nose breather. Head sags when not supported. Back rounded in sitting position. Hands held in fists. Can turn head to side when prone. Makes crawling movements when prone.	Cries when uncomfortable. Makes low throaty sounds.	SENSORIMOTOR PHASE *Reflective stage* Egocentric No intentionality; no expectations.	Regards faces intently.
2 months	Posterior fontanel closes. Can lift head 45 degrees when prone.	Crying differentiated. Coos. Vocalizes.	*Primary circular reactions stage* Responds differently to different objects.	May smile socially.

	When supported in sitting position, head is held up but bobs forward. Visually pursues objects and sounds. Hands held open more. Grasp reflex fading.	Voluntarily repeats activities, thereby demonstrating beginning connection between action and result. Anticipates feeding. Begins to separate self from others.	Squeals. Laughs. Vocalizes in response to other voices.	As for 2 months.
3 months	Holds hands in front and stares at them. Holds rattle but does not reach for it. Raises chest, supported on forearms. Little head lag. Visually pursues sound by turning head. Able to bear some weight on legs when held in standing position. Palmar grasp reflex weakening.			Recognizes familiar face and unfamiliar situations. Stops crying when parent approaches.

Continued

Table 22-1 Summary of Normal Growth and Development—cont'd

Age	Physical/Motor	Language	Cognition	Socialization
4 months	Holds head steady in sitting position. Almost no head lag when pulled to sitting position. Sits erect if propped. Lifts head and shoulders 90 degrees when prone. Turns from back to side. Plays with hands. Reaches for objects but overshoots. Grasps objects with both hands. Visually pursues objects that have been dropped. Begins drooling. Moro, tonic neck, extrusion, and rooting reflexes disappear. Sleeps 10-12 hours at night. Naps 2-3 times a day.	Makes consonant sounds (b, g, k, n, p) interspersed with vowel-like sounds. Vocalization varies with mood.	As for 2 months.	Sociable. Bored if left alone. Demands attention by fussing.

Age	Physical	Vocalization	Cognitive	Social
5 months	No head lag. Back straight when pulled to sitting. Bears most of weight on legs when standing. Sits for longer periods if back supported. Plays with feet. Takes objects to mouth at will. Teeth may begin to erupt.	As for 4 months.	*Secondary circular reactions stage* Searches for objects at point of disappearance. Recognizes partially hidden objects. Repeats interesting actions. Wide repertoire of activities (kicking, batting, pulling, patting) that produce novel results. Imitates others.	Recognizes strangers. May have rapid mood swings. Vocalizes displeasure if preferred object is taken.
6 months	Average weekly weight gain 90-150 gm (3-5 oz) for next 6 months. Chews and bites. May hold own bottle but prefers it to be held. Lifts chest and abdomen off flat surface, bearing weight on hands.	Vocalizes to mirror. Makes one-syllable sounds (ma, da, uh). Begins to mimic sounds (e.g., coughing).	As for 5 months.	Shows fear of strangers. Holds out arms when wants to be picked up. Becomes excited when familiar persons approach.

Continued

Table 22-1   Summary of Normal Growth and Development—cont'd

Age	Physical/Motor	Language	Cognition	Socialization
6 months— cont'd	Sits in highchair with back straight. Can turn completely from stomach to back to stomach. Picks up objects that have been dropped. Manipulates small objects. Pulls feet to mouth. Adjusts posture to visually pursue an object. Exhibits Landau reflex (when held prone, head raises and spine and legs extend).			Laughs when head covered with towel.
7 months	Sits in tripod position. Lifts head off table if supine. Bounces if held in standing position. Transfers cube from hand to hand. Holds cube in each hand.	Chains syllables (mama, dada) but does not attach meaning. Is able to produce four distinct vowel sounds.	As for 5 months.	Increasing fear of strangers. Imitative. Coughs, snorts to attract attention.

Bangs cube on table. Rakes at small objects. Can approach toy and grasp it with one hand. Responds to own name. Evidences taste preferences.			Closes lips in response to dislike of food. Bites and mouths. Plays peek-a-boo.
8 months	Sits alone steadily. May stand holding onto something. Beginning pincer (thumb-finger) grasp. Regards a third cube while holding a cube in each hand. Releases objects voluntarily. Rings bell purposely. Reaches for toys out of reach. May have night awakenings. Patterns emerge in bowel and bladder elimination.	Makes d, t, w sounds. Responds to simple commands.	As for 5 months. Coordination of secondary schemes. Object permanence.	Increased stranger anxiety and fear of separation from parent. Begins to respond to "no-no." Searches for hidden objects. Shows interest in pleasing parent.

Continued

Table 22-1   Summary of Normal Growth and Development—cont'd

Age	Physical/Motor	Language	Cognition	Socialization
9 months	Pulls self to standing position. Crawls, perhaps backward at first. Recovers sitting position if leaning forward, but cannot do so if leaning sideways.		Beginning of intelligence. Assigns symbols to events. Goal-directed activities.	May show fear of going to bed or of being alone.
10 months	Crawls, pulling self forward by hands. Stands holding onto furniture. May cruise (step sideways holding onto furniture). Recovers balance readily if sitting.	Comprehends dada, mama. May say one word.	As for 9 months.	Waves bye-bye. Extends toys to others but does not release toy. Repeats activities that attract attention. Plays pat-a-cake. Cries when scolded.
11 months	Creeps with abdomen off floor. Pivots when sitting (reaches backward to pick up an object).	Imitates speech sounds.	As for 9 months.	Expresses frustration when restricted.

Age	Physical / Fine Motor	Language		Social
	Intentionally drops objects for them to be picked up. Places objects inside each other. Holds crayon to make mark on paper.			Plays so-big, up-down, peek-a-boo.
12 months	Birth weight tripled. Head and chest circumference equal. Cruises well. Walks with help. Can sit from standing without help. Drinks from cup and eats from spoon but requires help. Cooperates in dressing. Neat pincer grasp. Turns several pages of book at a time. Lumbar nerve develops, with resulting lordosis when walking.	Says two or more words in addition to mama and dada. Recognizes objects by name. Imitates sounds of animals.	As for 9 months.	Responds to simple commands. Explores actively. Clings to mother in unfamiliar situations. May take security objects. Shows emotions.

Continued

Table 22-1   Summary of Normal Growth and Development—cont'd

Age	Physical/Motor	Language	Cognition	Socialization
13-18 months	Anterior fontanel closes. Abdomen protrudes. Walks with wide-based gait. Walks up stairs with help, creeps down stairs. Throws ball overhand. Seats self on small chair. Climbs. Pulls toys behind and pushes light furniture. Imitates housework. Puts shaped objects into holes. Scribbles vigorously. Imitates vertical and circular strokes. Builds tower of two or three cubes. Sleeps 10-12 hours. Has one afternoon nap. May uncover self during sleep.	By 15 months, infant able to say four to six words, and by 18 months, 10 words or more. Points to desired object. Points to two or three body parts (18 months).	*Tertiary circular reactions stage* Trial and error learning. Active experimentation. Solicits help of adults to bring about results. Understands relationship between object and use.	Drinks well from cup but may drop it when finished. Holds cup well in both hands. Uses spoon but turns bowl of spoon downward before it reaches mouth. May discard bottle. Less fearful of strangers. Hugs and kisses significant others and pictures in a book.

| 24 months | Average yearly weight gain 1.8-2.7 kg (4-6 lb). Chest circumference larger than head circumference. Physiologic systems stable except for reproductive and endocrine systems. Gait steadier, more adult. Jumps crudely. May pedal tricycle. Walks up and down stairs with two feet on each step. Holds onto rail. Picks up objects without falling. | Approximately 300 words in vocabulary. Short sentences of two or three words. Uses pronouns. Gives first name. Verbalizes need for food, drink, and toilet. | Inventions of new means through mental combinations. Beginning of mental problem solving and play. Has insight, forethought. Able to delay imitation for several days. | Temper tantrums begin. Beginning sense of ownership. Takes off simple clothes. Dawdles. Negativistic. Temper tantrums decrease. Treats other children as objects. Wants to make friends but doesn't know how. Cannot share possessions. Engages in parallel play. |

Continued

Table 22-1   Summary of Normal Growth and Development—cont'd

Age	Physical/Motor	Language	Cognition	Socialization
24 months—cont'd	Kicks ball forward without overbalancing. Turns doorknob and unscrews lids. Builds tower of six or seven cubes. Turns pages of book one at a time.			Shows increased independence from mother. Chews with mouth closed. Uses straw. Puts on simple clothing.
30 months	May be daytime toilet trained. Birth weight gain quadrupled. Primary dentition complete. Builds tower of eight cubes. Copies circle from model. Throws large ball 1.2-1.5 m (4-5 ft). Takes a few steps on tiptoe.	Gives first and last names. Enjoys rhymes and singing.	PREOPERATIONAL PHASE *Preconceptual stage* Symbols increasingly used. Egocentric. Representative thought. Symbolic and fantasy play. Beginning to understand concept of time.	Separates more easily from parent. Notices sex difference. Independent in toileting except for wiping.

| 36 months | Average yearly weight gain 1.8-2.7 kg (4-6 lb). Balances on one foot for 5 seconds. Jumps from a low step. Walks upstairs, alternating feet. May attempt to dance but balance still insecure. Pours fluid well from a pitcher. Begins to use scissors. Strings large beads. Builds tower of 9 or 10 cubes. Copies cross (X) from model. Washes hands. May be nighttime toilet trained. Sleeps 10-15 hours. Takes fewer naps. | Vocabulary of about 900 words. Talks in sentences of about six words. Uses telegraphic speech. Asks many questions. | Repeats three numbers. Remainder as for 30 months. | Less negativistic. Friendly. Begins to understand taking turns. Able to share but uses "mine" often. Begins to learn meaning of simple rules, but rules subject to own interpretation. Names appropriate sex of other. Boys tend to identify more strongly with father. |

Continued

Table 22-1   Summary of Normal Growth and Development—cont'd

Age	Physical/Motor	Language	Cognition	Socialization
36 months—cont'd				May dress with minimal assistance. Feeds self completely. Begins to use fork but holds it in fist. Uses adult form of chewing. May have fears, especially of dark or animals.
48 months	Length at birth doubled. Balances on one foot for 10 seconds. Hops on one foot. Catches bounced ball. Laces shoes. Imitates bridge with cubes.	Vocabulary of 1500 words. Knows simple songs. Exaggerates, boasts, may be mildly profane.	*Intuitive stage* Time linked with daily events. Counts but does not clearly understand what numbers mean.	Tattles. May have imaginary playmate. Independent. Aggressive. Takes out aggression on family members.

Age				
	Uses scissors to cut out picture. Immunoglobulin G reaches adult levels. Draws man in three parts.	Understands concepts of under, on top of, beside, in front of. Understands simple analogies.	Believes thoughts cause events. Cannot conserve matter. Egocentricism decreases. Repeats four numbers. Names one or more coins.	Exhibits mood swings. Engages in cooperative group play. Enjoys entertaining. Do's and don'ts important. Identifies with parent of opposite sex.
5 years	Permanent dentition may begin. Handedness established. Jumps rope. Walks backward heel-to-toe. May be able to tie shoelaces. Can form some letters correctly.	Vocabulary of about 2100 words. Talks constantly. Asks meanings of words.	Uses time words with more comprehension. Interested in facts associated with environment.	Comfortable. Trustworthy. Fewer fears. Eager to do things the right way.

Continued

Table 22-1 Summary of Normal Growth and Development—cont'd

Age	Physical/Motor	Language	Cognition	Socialization
5 years—cont'd	May print first name. Draws man in six or seven parts. Uses scissors or pencil well. Copies triangle and diamond.		Names four or more colors. Names coins. Names days of week.	May seek out mother more often because of more outside activities such as school. Identifies strongly with parent of same sex.
6 years	Dexterity increasing. Jumps rope. Skates, rides bicycle. May sew crudely.	Describes objects in pictures.	Knows right from left. Recognizes many shapes. Reads from memory. Obeys three commands in succession.	Enjoys bossing others. May be defiant and rude. Jealousy of younger siblings more apparent. May have temper tantrums. Cheats to win. Enjoys table games.

7 years	Increased speed and smoothness in motor activities. Uses common tools such as hammer and household utensils. More individual variation in skills.	Mechanical in reading. May skip words such as he, it.	Enjoys teasing. Girls play with girls, and boys with boys. Modest about sexual matters. Anxious over failures. Occasional periods of shyness or sadness. Increasing interest in spiritual matters.
		Repeats three numbers backward. Reads time to quarter hour.	
8-9 years		*Concrete operational stage (7-11 years)* Age of relational thinking. Able to classify, seriate, arrange in hierarchies.	Expansive. Wants to become involved in everything. Actively seeks company of others.

Continued

Table 22-1   Summary of Normal Growth and Development—cont'd

Age	Physical/Motor	Language	Cognition	Socialization
8-9 years— cont'd			Learns principle of conservation. Knows date. Gives days of week and months in order. Counts backward from 20 to 1. Makes change correctly from a quarter.	Likes clubs and fads. Hero worship begins. Likes to help. May reject Santa Claus, Easter Bunny. May show lack of interest in God.
10-12 years	Slow increase in height. Rapid increase in weight. Body changes associated with puberty may appear. Remainder of teeth erupt. Cooks, sews, paints, draws. Washes and dries own hair.	Likes writing letters. Reads for enjoyment or practical purposes.	FORMAL OPERATIONAL PHASE Logical thinking and ability to use abstract thought develops. Thinking is reflective, futuristic, multidimensional.	Very interested in reading, science, creative endeavors. Demonstrative. Peers and parents important. Conversational. Beginning interest in opposite sex.

| Early adolescence | Maximum increase in height, weight. Girls may commence menses. Girls may look more obese. May be clumsy and have poor posture. May have fatigue. Immunoglobulins A and M reach adult levels. | Spends long periods on telephone. | Clumsy and inconsistent in abstract thinking. Low point in creativity. | Differences intolerable. Conforms to group standards. Tries on various roles. Ambivalent. Mood swings. Period of intense conflict with parents. Boys gravitate toward sports. Girls discuss clothes, makeup. Daydreams a great deal. |

Continued

Table 22-1   Summary of Normal Growth and Development—cont'd

Age	Physical/Motor	Language	Cognition	Socialization
Middle adolescence	Girls reach physical maturity.	Able to maintain an argument.	Increased capacity for abstract reasoning. Enjoys intellectual powers. Concerned with philosophic and social problems. Creative period.	Introspective. Emotions still labile. Parent-child relationship may reach low point. Disengagement from dependent parent-child relationship occurs. Fears rejection by peers. Adheres to group norms. Sexual preference becoming established. Dating becomes important

| Late adolescence | Boys reach physical maturity. | Complex thinking. Creativity fading. | Pursues career. Sexual identity established. More comfortable with self. Fewer conflicts with family. Peer group less important. Emotions more controlled. Forms stable relationships. |

Assessment of Child Abuse 23

Rationale

Although the exact number of cases of child abuse and neglect is difficult to determine because of problems in identification and reporting, estimates place the incidence of child abuse and neglect in the United States at approximately 2.2 million cases annually. Minimally, 4,000 children die annually of abuse and neglect. The preeminence of abuse and neglect necessitates that nurses be alert to specific maltreatment indicators when assessing children.

Development of Abuse

Child abuse, defined as physical, psychological, sexual, or social injury damage, maltreatment, or corruption of a child, can be traced to parents, siblings, relatives, friends, professionals, and others who encounter the child. *Neglect* usually refers to intentional or unintentional failure to supply a child with the basic necessities of life.

Familial violence/abuse is generally considered to be the way in which a family system expresses its dysfunction. These families, which demonstrate several common characteristics (Table 23-1), may be geographically and emotionally isolated and may tend to discount, deny, or be unaware of the seriousness of their problems. Several factors (see box on page 296) can place a family at risk for violence and abuse, and awareness of these factors can assist the nurse in assessing families at all stages in family development.

Assessment of Abuse/Neglect in Children

Assessment of abuse and neglect should be ongoing and an integral part of a total health assessment. Findings that indicate abuse (see

Table 23-1   Characteristics of Abusive and Violent Families

Characteristic	Manifestations
Boundary	Rigid and inflexible. Little contact with outside social support systems. Within the family, there may be blurring of generational boundaries so that a daughter, for example, takes on the role of adult female sexual partner. Parent may seek gratification from child.
Affective tone	Helplessness, crisis, anger, powerlessness, depression. Competition for caring. Little empathy or evidence of nurturance, caring.
Control	Caring confused with conflict and abuse. Imbalance in power, often male or adult dominated. Members facilitate victim roles.
Instrumental functioning	Confusion about roles. Adult and child roles may be reversed. Intense attention to tasks or ineffective performance of tasks. Inappropriate age-related expectations of children.
Communication	Poor; double messages; mixed messages. Threats, sarcasm, blaming, demeaning communication. Incongruence in communication. Lack of meaningful communication. Family secrets common.
Role stereotyping	Traditionalist. Rigid. Role confusion, blurring, and reversal. Parental coalition limited or absent.

box on pp. 297-299) must be clearly documented and reported. Sexual abuse is more likely to be seen with girls; severe physical abuse with boys. Firstborns are more likely to be abused than those born later and children with disabilities are at risk for abuse. Care must be taken to describe, not interpret, behaviors and communications. In assessing for abuse, it is important to accurately describe findings and to be alert to whether reports of injury are congruent with child's age (e.g., a newborn cannot roll across a bed) and the events. If a child indicates that abuse has occurred, the

Factors That Place Families At Risk for Child Abuse and Neglect

History of childhood abuse, neglect, deprivation in parent(s)
Decreased knowledge of parenting skills and normal child development
Parental age at time of child's birth younger than 18 years
Level of parental education less than 12 years
Marital discord
Interspousal violence
Parental separation
Parent living alone or in unstable relationship
Unstable socioeconomic conditions
History of parental substance abuse/chemical dependency within last 6 months
Depression or emotional illness of mother during pregnancy or of parents
Violent older siblings
Chronically ill parent(s)
Parental substance abuse
Diminished self-esteem in parent(s)
Blended family
Prematurity of infant(s)
Developmental delays in child(ren)
Social isolation
Illegitimacy

child's report must be accepted and the child must be shown acceptance. Further exploration of abuse in the younger child can be facilitated by trained professionals through play, particularly through drawings and dramatic activities.

Related Nursing Diagnoses

Activity intolerance: Related to fatigue; inadequate intake of protein and calories.
Impaired verbal communication: Verbal related to fear, dysfunctional family relationships, social isolation, denial.

Indicators of Abuse and Neglect in Children

Emotional Abuse and Neglect

Failure to thrive (feeding difficulties, abnormally low height and weight, hypotonia, delayed dentition, developmental delays, passivity, self-stimulation behaviors)

Feeding disorders (rumination, anorexia)

Speech disorders

Enuresis

Sleep disorders

Psychosomatic complaints (headaches, nausea, abdominal pain)

Self-stimulation behaviors (rocking, head-banging, sucking)

Lack of stranger anxiety (infancy)

Withdrawal, indifference

Inhibition of play

Antisocial behavior (stealing, cruelty, destructiveness)

Suicide attempts

Physical Abuse and Neglect

Bruises and welts (on soft tissue areas such as buttocks, mouth, thighs, or torso; may be in various stages of healing; shape of bruises may approximate fingers, blunt objects). Differentiate bruises from mongolian spots (areas of deep blue pigmentation in sacral and gluteal areas; found in infants of Native American, African, Asian, or Hispanic descent); café-au-lait spots (pale tan macules); and bruises related to bleeding disorders (occur with minimal trauma over bony points).

Burns (may be friction, immersion, or pattern burns; located on soles of feet, hands, buttocks, back. Cigarette burns are round; immersion burns have lines of demarcation).

Fractures (multiple; various stages of healing; spiral fractures; fractures of skull, face, nose, ribs, and long bones more common)

Lacerations and abrasions (especially found on backs of arms, legs, torso, external genitalia, face, mouth, lips, or gums; human bite marks may be evident)

Whiplash

Chemical injuries (unexplained poisoning or illness)

Continued

Indicators of Abuse and Neglect in Children—cont'd

Failure to thrive, weight gain below normal (infants)
Signs of malnutrition (thinness, abdominal distention)
Unattended needs (glasses, dental work, physical injuries, immunization)
Poor physical hygiene (severe diaper rash, dirty hair, persistent body odor)
Unclean or inappropriate dress
Frequent accidents due to neglect
Unusual wariness or fear of adults
Withdrawal and/or lack of reaction
Inappropriate displays of friendliness and affection
Acting out (hitting, punching, biting, vandalism or shoplifting)
Absenteeism from school
Arriving early at school and staying late
Dullness, lethargy, inactivity
Begging and stealing food
Consistent lack of supervision

Sexual Abuse

Bruises, bleeding, fissures, or lacerations of external genitalia, vagina, or anus
Abnormalities of hymen
Labial fusion
Anal laxity, anal gaping
Swelling of scrotum/penis (sucking injury)
Bloody or stained underwear
Difficulty walking and/or sitting
Venereal disease in young child
Vaginal or penile discharge
Recurrent vaginal infections
Pain on urination
Persistent sore throats of unknown origin
Pregnancy in adolescent females
Withdrawal
Preoccupation with fantasies
Unusual or precocious sexual behavior and knowledge
Sudden changes in behavior (nightmares, fears, phobias, regression, acute anxiety)

Continued

Indicators of Abuse and Neglect in Children—cont'd

Noticeable personality changes
Anger at mother (in incestuous relationships)
Poor peer relationships
Infantile behaviors
Self-mutilation
Suicidal thoughts or attempts
Abuse of drugs or alcohol

Emotional Deprivation/Abuse

Excessive criticism by parent
Embarrassment of child by parent
Name calling by parent
Unresponsiveness or diminished responses to child's needs
    and interactions
Language delays
Anxiety, fear, diminished responsiveness, low
    self-confidence
Wetting/soiling
Poor school progress or changes in school performance
School truancy; school phobia
Runs away
Substance abuse
Stealing

Ineffective family coping: Related to family history of sexual abuse, multiple stressors, maturity of parents, childhood abuse or neglect of parents; violence in parental relationship.

Compromised family coping: Related to dysfunctional communication; violence.

Fear: Related to knowledge deficit, dysfunctional family relationships, violence, ridicule, criticism.

Delayed growth and development: Related to deficit of protein and calories; neglect; lack of emotional caring; decreased stimulation.

Ineffective health maintenance: Related to lack of knowledge; abuse; neglect; substance abuse; alcohol abuse.

Infection: Related to inappropriate sexual contact, injury.

Deficient knowledge: Related to normal development; community resources; support systems.

Impaired physical mobility: Secondary to abuse, neglect.

Imbalanced nutrition: Less than body requirements related to lack of knowledge of adequate nutrition; neglect; physical injury to face or abdomen.

Self-esteem: Disturbances in body image, role performance, personal identity related to dysfunctional family relationships; physical or sexual abuse.

Ineffective sexuality patterns: Related to abuse.

Skin integrity, impairment of: Related to neglect; physical or sexual abuse.

Impaired skin integrity: Related to burns, abrasions, cuts, penetration, infection.

Self-mutilation: Related to guilt, poor self-esteem, abuse.

CONCLUDING THE ASSESSMENT

V

Completing the Examination

24

- Signal to the child and the parent that the assessment is at an end.
- Provide an opportunity for the parent and child to ask questions or verbalize concerns.
- Assist the child to dress.
- Praise the child for cooperation during the examination. Offer reassurance and empathy to the child who has been frightened or upset.
- Express appreciation to the parent for assistance.
- Share assessment findings with the parent (and child, if appropriate). *If findings are abnormal, the beginning practitioner should confirm them with a more experienced nurse before sharing with the parents and child.*
- Findings that initiate concern for the *immediate welfare* of the child, such as respiratory difficulties and abnormal neurologic signs, should be *communicated directly and quickly* to the physician and appropriate health care providers.
- Findings should be organized and written down as soon as possible after assessment to avoid inaccurate or vague documentation of detail (see Appendix E).
- If unsure of the correct terminology, describe the findings.
- Avoid use of "good" and "normal." These terms are subjective and vary greatly from nurse to nurse. Use specific, descriptive terms. Measurements, where possible, should be included.
- Findings should be documented in a way that is organized, concise, specific, accurate, complete, confidential, and legible.

APPENDIXES

Developmental
Assessment

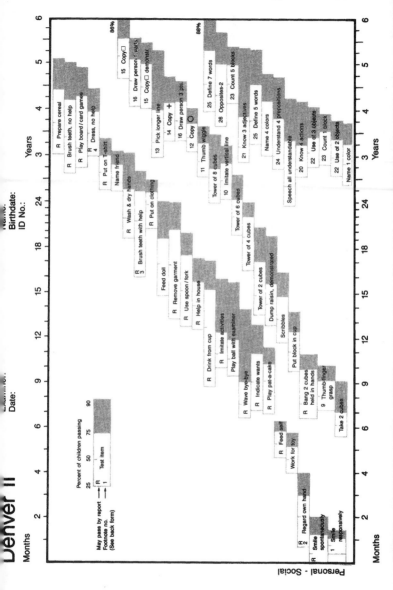

Figure A-1
Denver II.
(From WK Frankenburg and JB Dodds, University of Colorado Medical Center, 1990.)

Continued

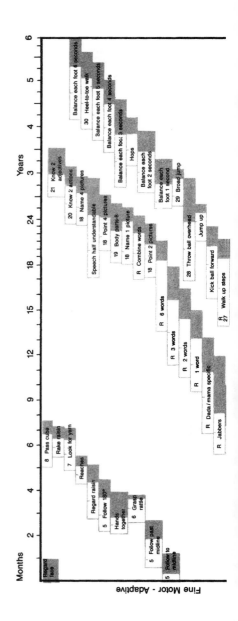

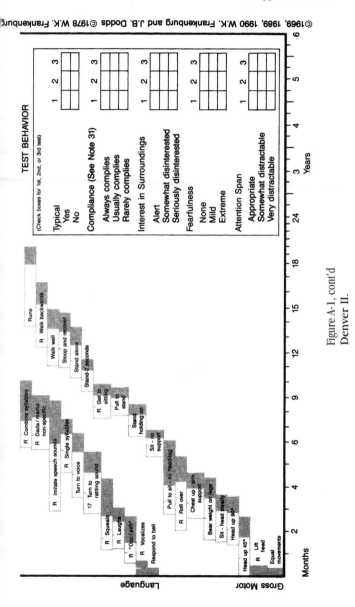

Figure A-1, cont'd
Denver II.

DIRECTIONS FOR ADMINISTRATION

1. Try to get child to smile by smiling, talking or waving. Do not touch him/her.
2. Child must stare at hand several seconds.
3. Parent may help guide toothbrush and put toothpaste on brush.
4. Child does not have to be able to tie shoes or button/zip in the back.
5. Move yarn slowly in an arc from one side to the other, about 8" above child's face.
6. Pass if child grasps rattle when it is touched to the backs or tips of fingers.
7. Pass if child tries to see where yarn went. Yarn should be dropped quickly from sight from tester's hand without arm movement.
8. Child must transfer cube from hand to hand without help of body, mouth, or table.
9. Pass if child picks up raisin with any part of thumb and finger.
10. Line can vary only 30 degrees or less from tester's line.
11. Make a fist with thumb pointing upward and wiggle only the thumb. Pass if child imitates and does not move any fingers other than the thumb.

12. Pass any enclosed form. Fail continuous round motions.

13. Which line is longer? (Not bigger.) Turn paper upside down and repeat. (pass 3 of 3 or 5 of 6)

14. Pass any lines crossing near midpoint.

15. Have child copy first. If failed, demonstrate.

16. When giving items 12, 14, and 15, do not name the forms. Do not demonstrate 12 and 14.
17. When scoring, each pair (2 arms, 2 legs, etc.) counts as one part.
18. Place one cube in cup and shake gently near child's ear, but out of sight. Repeat for other ear.

Figure A-2
Directions for administration of numbered items on Denver II.
(From WK Frankenburg and JB Dodds, University of Colorado Medical Center, 1990.)

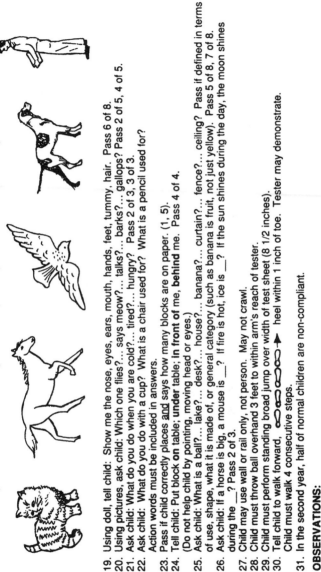

18. Point to picture and have child name it. (No credit is given for sounds only.)
If less than 4 pictures are named correctly, have child point to picture as each is named by tester.

19. Using doll, tell child: Show me the nose, eyes, ears, mouth, hands, feet, tummy, hair. Pass 6 of 8.
20. Using pictures, ask child: Which one flies?... says meow?... talks?... barks?... gallops? Pass 2 of 5, 4 of 5.
21. Ask child: What do you do when you are cold?... tired?... hungry? Pass 2 of 3, 3 of 3.
22. Ask child: What do you do with a cup? What is a chair used for? What is a pencil used for?
    Action words must be included in answers.
23. Pass if child correctly places <u>and</u> says how many blocks are on paper. (1, 5).
24. Tell child: Put block **on** table; **under** table; **in front of** me, **behind** me. Pass 4 of 4.
    (Do not help child by pointing, moving head or eyes.)
25. Ask child: What is a ball?... lake?... desk?... house?... banana?... curtain?... fence?... ceiling? Pass if defined in terms
    of use, shape, what it is made of, or general category (such as banana is fruit, not just yellow). Pass 5 of 8, 7 of 8.
26. Ask child: If a horse is big, a mouse is __? If fire is hot, ice is __? If the sun shines during the day, the moon shines
    during the __? Pass 2 of 3.
27. Child may use wall or rail only, not person. May not crawl.
28. Child must throw ball overhand 3 feet to within arm's reach of tester.
29. Child must perform standing broad jump over width of test sheet (8 1/2 inches).
30. Tell child to walk forward, 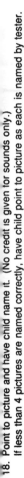 heel within 1 inch of toe. Tester may demonstrate.
    Child must walk 4 consecutive steps.
31. In the second year, half of normal children are non-compliant.

OBSERVATIONS:

Figure A-2, cont'd

Directions for administration of numbered items on Denver II.

Growth Charts

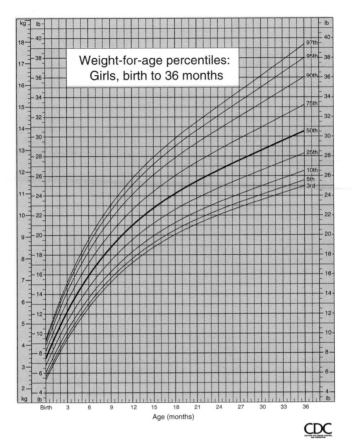

Figure B-1
Weight-for-age percentiles, girls, birth to 36 months,
CDC growth charts: United States.
(Developed by the National Center for Health Statistics in collaboration with the
National Center for Chronic Disease Prevention and Health Promotion, 2000.)

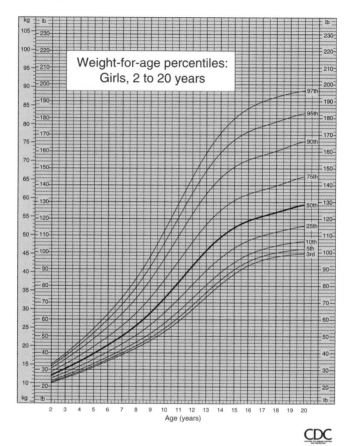

Figure B-2
Weight-for-age percentiles, girls, 2 to 20 years, CDC growth charts: United States.
(Developed by the National Center for Health Statistics in collaboration with the National Center for Chronic Disease Prevention and Health Promotion, 2000.)

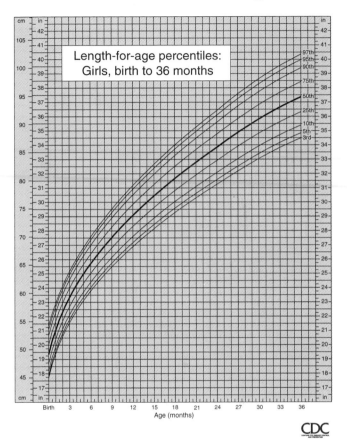

Figure B-3
Length-for-age percentiles, girls, birth to 36 months,
CDC growth charts: United States.
(Developed by the National Center for Health Statistics in collaboration with the
National Center for Chronic Disease Prevention and Health Promotion, 2000.)

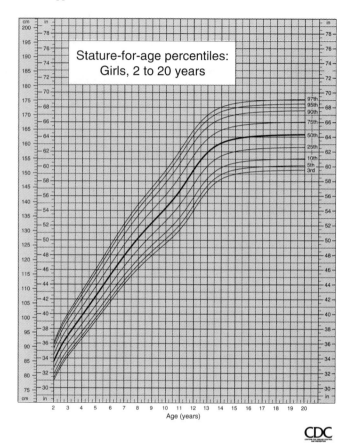

Figure B-4

Stature-for-age percentiles, girls, 2 to 20 years, CDC growth charts: United States.

(Developed by the National Center for Health Statistics in collaboration with the National Center for Chronic Disease Prevention and Health Promotion, 2000.)

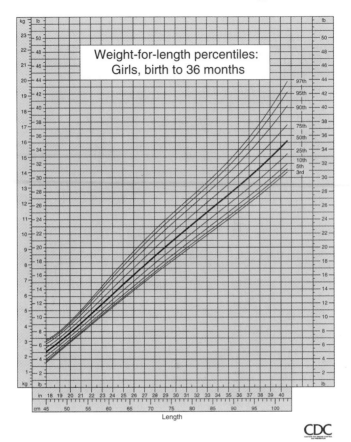

Figure B-5
Weight-for-length percentiles, girls, birth to 36 months, CDC growth charts: United States.
(Developed by the National Center for Health Statistics in collaboration with the National Center for Chronic Disease Prevention and Health Promotion, 2000.)

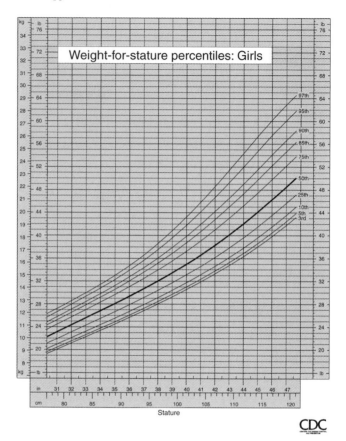

Figure B-6

Weight-for-stature percentiles, girls, CDC growth charts: United States.

(Developed by the National Center for Health Statistics in collaboration with the National Center for Chronic Disease Prevention and Health Promotion, 2000.)

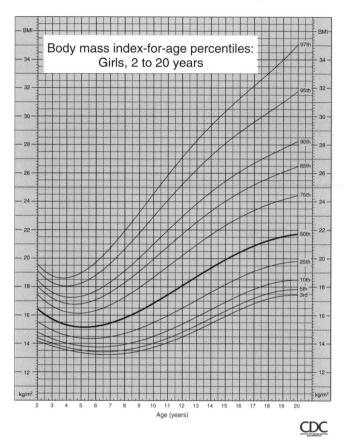

Figure B-7
Body mass index-for-age percentiles, girls, 2 to 20 years,
CDC growth charts: United States.
(Developed by the National Center for Health Statistics in collaboration with the
National Center for Chronic Disease Prevention and Health Promotion, 2000.)

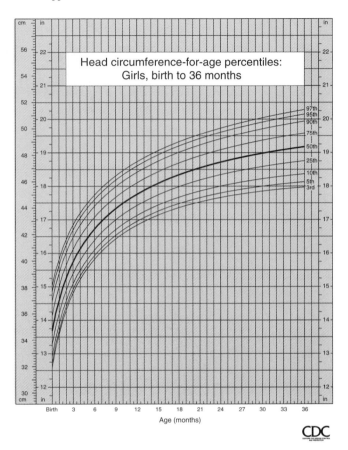

Figure B-8
Head circumference-for-age percentiles, girls, birth to
36 months, CDC growth charts: United States.
(Developed by the National Center for Health Statistics in collaboration with the
National Center for Chronic Disease Prevention and Health Promotion, 2000.)

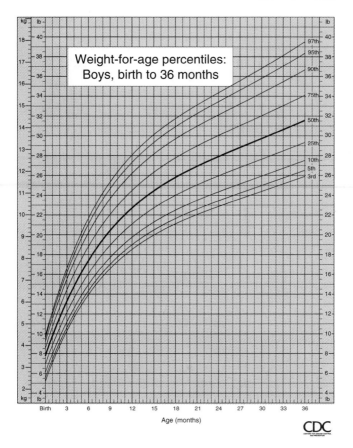

Figure B-9
**Weight-for-age percentiles, boys, birth to 36 months,
CDC growth charts: United States.**
(Developed by the National Center for Health Statistics in collaboration with the
National Center for Chronic Disease Prevention and Health Promotion, 2000.)

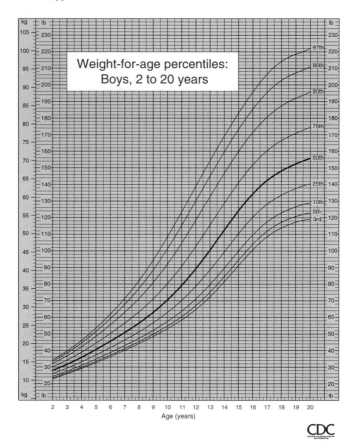

Figure B-10

Weight-for-age percentiles, boys, 2 to 20 years, CDC growth charts: United States.

(Developed by the National Center for Health Statistics in collaboration with the National Center for Chronic Disease Prevention and Health Promotion, 2000.)

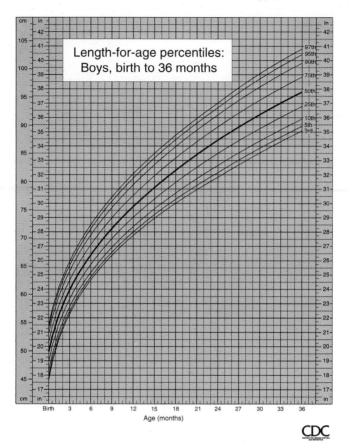

Figure B-11
Length-for-age percentiles, boys, birth to 36 months,
CDC growth charts: United States.
(Developed by the National Center for Health Statistics in collaboration with the
National Center for Chronic Disease Prevention and Health Promotion, 2000.)

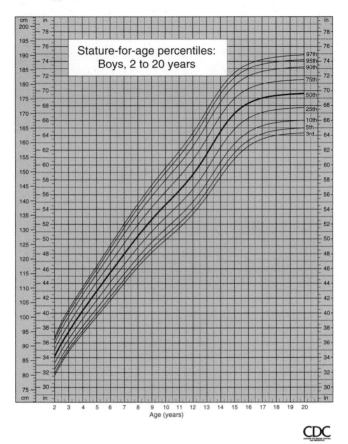

Figure B-12
Stature-for-age percentiles, boys, 2 to 20 years, CDC growth charts: United States.
(Developed by the National Center for Health Statistics in collaboration with the National Center for Chronic Disease Prevention and Health Promotion, 2000.)

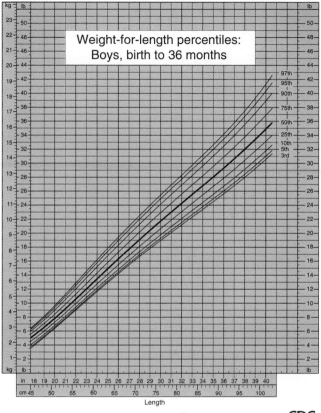

Weight-for-length percentiles:
Boys, birth to 36 months

CDC

Figure B-13
**Weight-for-length percentiles, boys, birth to 36 months,
CDC growth charts: United States.**
(Developed by the National Center for Health Statistics in collaboration with the
National Center for Chronic Disease Prevention and Health Promotion, 2000.)

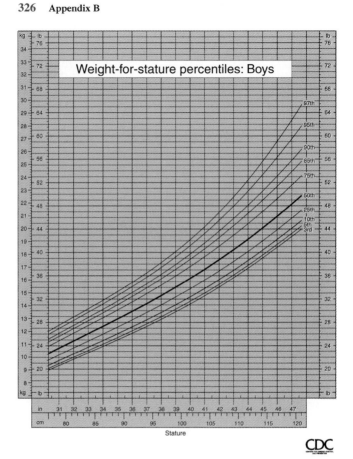

Figure B-14

Weight-for-stature percentiles, boys, CDC growth charts: United States.

(Developed by the National Center for Health Statistics in collaboration with the National Center for Chronic Disease Prevention and Health Promotion, 2000.)

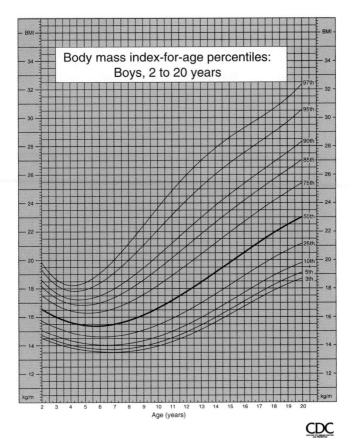

Figure B-15
Body mass index-for-age percentiles, boys, 2 to 20 years,
CDC growth charts: United States.
(Developed by the National Center for Health Statistics in collaboration with the
National Center for Chronic Disease Prevention and Health Promotion, 2000.)

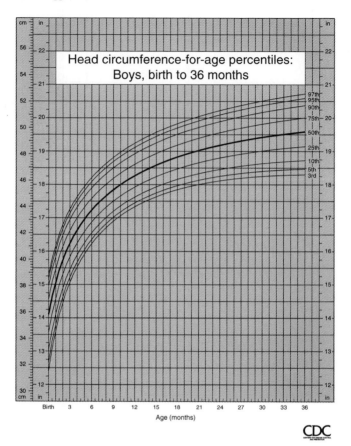

Figure B-16
Head circumference-for-age percentiles, boys, birth to
36 months, CDC growth charts: United States.
(Developed by the National Center for Health Statistics in collaboration with the
National Center for Chronic Disease Prevention and Health Promotion, 2000.)

Normal
Laboratory
Values

C

Table C-1 Hematology

Test	Age/Sex	Reference Range	
		Conventional Values	International Units
Hematocrit (Hct; HCT)		% Packed Cells	Volume Fraction
	Infant (2 mo)	28-42	0.28-0.42
	Child (6-12 yr)	35-45	0.35-0.45
	Adolescent: Male	37-49	0.37-0.49
	Female	36-46	0.36-0.46
	Panic levels	<15	<0.15
		>60	>0.60
Hemoglobin (Hb, Hgb)		gm/dl	mmol/L
	Infant (2-6 mo)	9-14	1.40-2.17
	Child (6-12 yr)	10-17	6.21-10.55
	Adolescent: Male	13-16	2.02-2.48
	Female	12-16	1.86-2.48
		Million	
		Cells/mm^3 (μL)	×10^{12} Cells/L
	Panic levels	<5	3.10
		>20	12.41

		Conventional	SI
Red blood cell count (erythrocyte count; RBC count)	Infant	3.8-6.1	3.8-6.1
	Child (2-12 yr)	3.6-5.5	3.6-5.5
	Adolescent: Male	4.7-6.1	4.7-6.1
	Female	4.1-5.4	4.1-5.4
		$\times 10^3/mm^3$ (μL)	$\times 10^9/L$
Platelet count (thrombocyte count)	Newborn	150-300	150-300
	Infant	200-475	200-475
	Child and thereafter	150-400	150-400
Blood indices			
Mean corpuscular volume (MCV)		μm^3	fL
	Infant	70-86	70-86
	Child (6-12 yr)	77-96	77-96
	Adolescent: Male (12-18 yr)	78-98	78-98
	Female (12-18 yr)	78-102	78-102
Mean corpuscular hemoglobin (MCH)		pg/Cell	fmol/Cell
	2-6 mo	25-35	0.39-0.54
	6-24 mo	23-31	0.36-0.48
	Thereafter	25-34	0.39-0.54
Mean corpuscular hemoglobin concentration (MCHC)		%Hb/Cell	mmol
	Infant	30-36	4.65-5.58
	Thereafter	31-37	4.81-5.74
		%	Number Fraction

Continued

Table C-1 Hematology—cont'd

Test	Age/Sex	Reference Range		
		Conventional Values	International Units
Blood indices—cont'd			
Reticulocyte count	Infant	0.3-3.1	0.003-0.031
	Thereafter	0.5-2.5	0.005-0.025
		mm/hr	mm/hr
Sedimentation rate (erythrocyte sedimentation rate or ESR)	Child	0-10	0-10
	Thereafter: Male	1-15	1-15
	Female	1-20	1-20
		× 1000 Cells/mm³ (μL)	×10⁹ Cells/L
White blood cell count (leukocyte count)	Newborn	9.0-30.0	9.0-30.0
	Child ≤2 years	6.2-17.0	6.2-17.0
	Child/adult	5.0-10.0	5.0-10.0
	Panic value	<2.5 or >30.0	
		%	Number Fraction
Differential white blood cell count			
Neutrophils (segmented and bands)	Infant	23	0.23
	Child	31-61	0.31-0.61
	Thereafter	54-75	0.54-0.75

		%	Number Fraction
Eosinophils		1-3	0.01-0.03
Basophils		0.5-1	0.005-0.01
Lymphocytes		61	0.61
	Infant	28-48	0.28-0.48
	Child	25-40	0.25-0.40
	Thereafter		
Monocytes		5	0.05
	Infant	4-4.5	0.04-0.045
	Child	2-8	0.02-0.08
	Thereafter		
Bleeding time	Infant/child/adolescent	2-7 min	2-7 min
	Critical value	>12 min	>12 min
Clotting time	Infant/child/adolescent	5-8 min	5-8 min
Prothrombin time (PT), one stage, quick	Infant/child/adolescent	11-15 sec	11-15 sec
Partial thromboplastin time (PTT), nonactivated	Infant/child/adolescent	24-40 sec	24-40 sec
Partial thromboplastin time (APTT), activated	Infant (to 6 mo)	<90 sec	<90 sec
	Thereafter	30-40 sec	30-40 sec
		mg/dl	
Fibrinogen level (Factor 1, Quantitative fibrinogen)	Infant/child/adolescent	200-400	2.00-4.0
	Critical values	<100	<100

Table C-2   Normal Cerebrospinal Fluid Values

Test	Age/Sex	Reference Range	
		Conventional Values	International Units
Appearance		Clear, colorless	
Chloride		mmol/L	mmol/L
	Infant/child/adolescent	118-132	118-132
Glucose		mg/dL	mmol/L
	Infant/child/adolescent	40-80 (fasting)	2.2-4.4 (fasting)
Differential leukocyte count		%	Number Fraction
Differential lymphocytes		63-99	0.63-0.99
Beta lymphocytes		0-4	0-0.04
T-lymphocytes		89-97	0.89-0.97
Leukocytes		0-10 µL	$0-10 \times 10^6$/L
Lymphocytes		62 ± 34	0.62 ± 0.34
Monocytes		3-37	0.03-0.37

Neutrophils	Absent	Absent
Eosinophils	0-5	0-0.05
	mg/dL	mg/L
Erythrocytes	0-10 µL	$0-10 \times 10^6$/L
Neoplastic cells	Negative	Negative
Pressure	50-175 mm H_2O	50-175 mm H_2O
WBC	0-10 mg/L	
Protein, total	15-45	150-450
	mmol/L	mmol/L
Sodium	138-154	138-154
Specific gravity	1.006-1.008	1.006-1.008

Table C-3 Blood Chemistry Values

Test	Specimen	Age/Sex	Reference Range Conventional Values	Reference Range International Units
Acetone	Serum/plasma		mg/dL	mmol/L
Semiquantitative			Negative	Negative
Quantitative			0.3-2.0	0.05-0.34
Alkaline phosphatase (King-Armstrong method)	Serum		u/dL	U/L
		Infant (1 mo)	10-30	71-213
		Toddler (3 yrs)	10-20	71-142
		Child (10 yrs)	15-30	107-213
		Adults	4.5-13	32-92
Amylase (Somogyi method)	Serum	Infant/child/adult	50-180 U/dL	92-330 U/L
	Urine (24 hr)	Infant/child/adult	26-950 U/24 hr	
Bilirubin			mg/dL	μmol/L
Total	Serum	Infant/child/adolescent	<1.5	1.7-20.5
Direct (conjugated)	Serum	Infant/child/adolescent	0.0-0.3	1.7-5.1

			mg/dL	mmol/L
Calcium				
Ionized	Serum, plasma whole blood	Infant/child/adolescent	4.48-4.92	1.12-2.70
Total	Serum	Child	8.8-10.8	2.2-2.70
		Thereafter	8.4-10.2	2.1-2.55
			μg/dL	μmol/L
β-Carotene	Serum	Infant	20-70	0.37-1.30
		Child	40-130	0.74-2.42
		Thereafter	60-200	1.12-3.72
			mEq/L	mmol/L
Chloride	Serum/plasma	Infant/child/adolescent	97-107	97-107
Panic levels			<80	<80
			>115	>115
Urine		Infant	2-10	2-10
		Child	15-40	15-40
		Adolescent	36-176	36-176
Sweat		Normal	5-45	5-45
		Marginal	45-70	45-70
		Cystic fibrosis	70-200	70-200
			mg/dL	mmol/L
Cholesterol, total	Serum*	Infant (≤4 yr)	112-203	2.9-5.25
		Child	121-205	3.13-5.30
		Adolescent	113-200	2.93-5.18

*Values for African-American are approximately 10% higher.

Continued

Table C-3 Blood Chemistry Values—cont'd

Test	Specimen	Age/Sex	Conventional Values	International Units
Copper	Serum	Infant/child	mg/dL 30-190	mmol/L 4.7-29.83
		Adolescent	70-155	10.99-24.34
Cortisol	Plasma, serum	Infant/child	μg/dL 5-23	nmol/L 138-635
		Adolescent	2-15	55-413
Creatine kinase (CK, CPK)	Serum	Infant/child/ adolescent: Male Female	U/L 0-70 0-50	U/L 0-70 0-50
		(higher in African Americans and after exercise)		
Creatinine	Serum, plasma	Infant Child Adolescent	mg/dL ≤0.5 ≤0.6-0.9 ≤1.1-1.2	μmol/L ≤44 ≤53-80 ≤97-106
Fatty acids, free	Serum, plasma	Children/obese adults	mg/dL <31 g/day	mmol/L <1.10 g/day

Fecal fat	Feces	Breast-fed infant	<1
		0-6 yr	<2
		Thereafter	<4
			θg/L
Ferritin	Serum	1 mo	200-600
		2-5 mo	50-200
		6 mo-15 yr	7-140
			nmol/L
Folate	Serum	Infant/child/adolescent	4.1-20.4
			mmol/L
Galactose	Serum	Infant/child/adolescent	<0.28
			mmol/L
Glucose	Serum	Child	3.3-5.5
		Adolescent	3.9-5.8
		Panic levels	<2.2
			>38.6
	Urine (qualitative)		Negative

Fecal fat	Feces	Breast-fed infant	<1
		0-6 yr	<2
		Thereafter	<4
			ng/ml
Ferritin	Serum	1 mo	200-600
		2-5 mo	50-200
		6 mo-15 yr	7-140
			ng/ml
Folate	Serum	Infant/child/adolescent	1.8-9
			mg/dL
Galactose	Serum	Infant/child/adolescent	<5
			mg/dL
Glucose	Serum	Child	60-100
		Adolescent	70-105
		Panic levels	<40
			>700
	Urine (qualitative)		Negative

Continued

Table C-3 Blood Chemistry Values—cont'd

Test	Specimen	Age/Sex		Reference Range			
				Conventional Values		International Units	
			mg/dL Normal	mg/dL Diabetic		mmol/L Normal	mmol/L Diabetic
Glucose tolerance (GTT)		Time (min)					
		Fasting	70-105	>115		3.9-5.8	>6.4
		60	120-160	>200		6.7-8.8	≥11
		90	100-140	>200		5.6-7.8	≥11
		120	65-120	>140		3.6-6.7	≥7.8
Dosage							
0-18 mo	2.5 gm/kg						
18 mo-3 yr	2.0 gm/kg						
3-12 yr	1.75 gm/kg						
>12 yr	1.25 gm/kg (maximum 100 gm)						
				mg/day		µmol/day	
17-Hydroxycorticosteroids (17-OHCS)	Urine 24 hr	Infant		0.5-1.0		1.4-2.8	
		Child		1.0-5.6		2.8-15.5	
		Adolescent: Male		3.0-10.0		8.2-27.6	
		Female		2.0-8.0		5.5-22	

Immunoglobulin A (IgA)	Serum		mg/dL	g/L
		1-6 mo	7-46	0.07-0.46
		6 mo-2 yr	19-74	0.19-0.74
		3-5 yr	66-120	0.66-1.20
		6-11 yr	71-191	0.71-1.91
		12-16 yr	85-211	0.85-2.11
Immunoglobulin D (IgD)	Serum		mg/dL	µmol/L
		Child/adolescent	0-8	5-30
Immunoglobulin E (IgE)	Serum		IU/mL	µg/L
		6 wk	0.1-2.8	0.24-9.6
		6 mo	0.9-28	0.24-134.4
		1 yr	1.1-10.2	0.24-199.2
		4 yr	2.4-34.8	0.96-345.6
		10 yr	0.3-215	4.56-1010.4
		14 yr	1.9-159	3.84-1094.0
Immunoglobulin G (IgG)	Serum		mg/dL	g/L
		1-6 mo	250-900	2.5-9
		6 mo-2 yr	220-1070	2.2-10.7
		2-6 yr	420-1200	4.2-12.0
		>6 yr	650-1600	6.5-16.0

Continued

Table C-3   Blood Chemistry Values—cont'd

Test	Specimen	Age/Sex	Reference Range	
			Conventional Values	International Units
Iron	Serum		µg/dL	µmol/L
		Infant	40-100	7.16-17.90
		Child	50-120	8.95-21.48
		Adolescent: Male	50-160	8.95-28.64
		Female	40-150	7.16-26.85
		Intoxicated child	280-2550	50.12-456.5
		Fatally poisoned child	>1800	322.2
Iron-binding capacity	Serum		µg/dL	µmol/L
		Infant	100-400	17.90-71.60
		Thereafter	250-400	44.75-71.60
Lead	Whole blood		µg/dL	µmol/L
		Child	<10	<0.5
		Adult	<20	<1.0
		Lead encephalopathy in children	≥100	>4.8
Lipase (Tietz method)	Serum	Child/adolescent	µg/dL 0.1-1.0	µmol/L 28-280

Analyte	Specimen	Age/Condition	Conventional Units	SI Units
Magnesium	Serum	Infant/child/adolescent	mEq/L 1.3-2.1	mmol/L 0.65 ± 1.05
Osmolality	Serum		mOsm/kg H_2O 275-295	mmol/L
Phenylalanine	Serum	Infant/child/adolescent	mg/dL 0.8-1.8	mmol/L 0.05-0.11
Phenylketonuria	Serum	Infant negative or <3 mg/dL		
Phosphorus, inorganic	Serum	Infant/child Adolescent	mg/dL 4.5-6.5 3.0-4.5 mmol/L	mmol/L 1.45-2.1 0.97-1.45 mmol/L
Potassium	Serum	Infant Child Adolescent	4.1-5.3 3.4-4.7 3.5-5.3	4.1-5.3 3.4-4.7 3.5-5.3
Protein, total	Serum	Child Adolescent	g/dL 6.2-8.0 6.0-8.0	g/L 62.0-80.0 60.0-80.0
Salicylates	Serum, plasma	Therapeutic Toxic	mg/dL 15-30 >30	mmol/L 1.1-2.2 >2.2

Continued

Table C-3 Blood Chemistry Values—cont'd

Test	Specimen	Age/Sex	Reference Range Conventional Values	Reference Range International Units
Sodium	Serum	Infant	mmol/L 139-146	mmol/L 139-146
		Child	138-145	138-145
		Adolescent	135-148	135-148
Thiamine (vitamin B$_1$)	Whole blood		μg/dL 0-2.0	nmol/L 0.75-4
Thyroid-stimulating hormone (hTSH)	Serum, plasma	Infant/child/adolescent	μU/L 2-11	μU/L 2-11
Transferrin	Serum	Infant/child/adolescent	mg/dL 200-400	g/L 2.0-4.0
Triglycerides (TG: neutral fat)	Serum	Infant	mg/dL 5-40	g/L 0.05-0.40
		Adolescent	30-150	0.30-1.50
		Male	40-160	0.40-1.60
		Female	35-135	0.35-1.35

	Specimen	Category	Conventional Units	SI Units
Tyrosine	Serum	Infant/child/adolescent	mg/dL 0.8-1.3	mmol/L 0.044-0.07
Urea nitrogen	Serum, plasma	Infant/child Adolescent	mg/dL 5-18 7-18	mmol urea/L 1.8-6.4 2.5-6.4
Uric acid	Serum	Child Adolescent: Male Female	mg/dL 2.0-5.5 3.5-7.2 3.0-8.2	μmol/L 119-327 208-438 178-488
Vitamin A	Serum	Child Adolescent	μm/dL 30-80 30-65	μmol/L 1.22-2.62 1.05-2.27
Vitamin B_{12}	Serum	Infant/child/adolescent	pg/ml 140-900	pmol/L 103-454
Vitamin C	Serum	Infant/child/adolescent	mg/dL 0.6-2.0	μmol/L 34-113
Vitamin E	Serum	Infant/child	μg/mL 5-20	μmol/L 17.6-46.4

Table C-4 Blood Gas Determinations

Determination	Age	Reference Range	
		Conventional Values	International Units
pH	Infant 2 mo-2 yr	7.34-7.46	7.34-7.46
	Child (over 2 yr)	7.35-7.45	7.35-7.45
	Panic values	<7.2	<7.2
		≥7.6	≥7.6
		mmHg	k/Pa
P_{CO_2}	Child/adolescent	35-45	4.7-6.0
	Panic values	≤20	<2.7
		>70	>9.4
Pao_2	Child/adolescent	75-100	10.0-13.3
	Panic values	≤10 mEq/L	<10 mmol/L
		mmol/L	mmol/L
Hco_3, venous	Infant/child/adolescent (arterial approximately 2 mmol/L lower)	22-26	22-26
	Panic values	>40	>40
		mEq/L	mmol/L
Base excess	Infant	(−7)-(−1)	(−7)-(−1)
	Child	(−4)-(+2)	(−4)-(+2)
	Thereafter	(−3)-(+3)	(−3)-(+3)
O_2 saturation	Child/adolescent	96-100%	0.96-1.00
	Panic value	≤60%	<0.60

Table C-5 Urinalysis

Test	Age/Sex	Reference Range	
		Conventional Values	International Units
Bilirubin		Negative	Negative
Colony count	Infant/child	Clean catch	Catheterization
		<1000	100
	Thereafter	<10,000	100
Glucose, qualitative		Negative	Negative
Microscopy		Per high-power field	
Leukocytes		0-4	
Erythrocytes		Rare	
Casts		Rare	
Occult blood		Negative	Negative
Osmolality		mOsm/kg H$_2$O	
Random	Infant/child/adolescent	50-1400	
24-Hour	Infant/child/adolescent	300-900	
		μmol/L	μmol/L
pH	Infant/child/adolescent	4.5-8	0.01-32.0

Immunization Schedules for Infants and Children

D

Table D-1   Recommended Immunization Schedule for Infants and Children (2000)

Age	Immunization	Comments
Birth	HBV	Hepatitis B vaccine is given to mothers who are hepatitis B positive. The third dose should be administered at least 4 months after the first dose and at least 2 months after the second dose.
1-2 mo	HBV	
2 mo	DTaP	Diphtheria, tetanus toxoids, and acellular pertussis vaccine is the preferred vaccine for all doses in the vaccination series. Whole-cell DTP is an acceptable alternative to DTaP. Children younger than 7 years may experience localized redness, swelling, and tenderness at the injection site. Fever is common in the first 12-24 hours.
	IPV	Inactivated polio vaccine. IPV is also recommended and acceptable for children who are immunocompromised and their household contacts.
	Hib	*Haemophilus influenzae* B conjugate (vaccine). Types of vaccine are licensed for infant use. If PRP-OMP is used, a third dose at 6 months is not required. DtaP/Hib combination products should not be used for primary vaccination in young infants unless approved for these ages.
4 mo	DTaP, Hib, IPV	
6 mo	Hib (depending on type of vaccine)	

American Academy of Pediatrics, American Academy of Family Physicians: Recommended childhood immunization schedule United States, January-December 2000.

Continued

Table D-1   Recommended Immunization Schedule for Infants and Children (2000)—cont'd

Age	Immunization	Comments
6-18 mo	IPV HBV Hib	
12-15 mo	MMR	Live attenuated measles-mumps-rubella vaccine. May produce fever, rash 10-14 days after administration.
12-18 mo	DTaP Varicella	Varicella can be given at any visit after the first birthday to susceptible children (i.e., those who have not been vaccinated and those who lack a reliable history of having had the disease).
4-6 yr	DTaP IPV MMR	
11-12 yr	Td	Tetanus-diphtheria toxoids. Can be given at 11-12 years of age if at least 5 years have elapsed since last dose of DTaP, DPT, or DT. Subsequent boosters recommended every 10 years.
11-12 yr	HBV MMR Varicella	These vaccines are given if previously recommended doses missed or if doses given earlier than recommended ages.

American Academy of Pediatrics, American Academy of Family Physicians: Recommended childhood immunization schedule United States, January-December 2000.

Sample Documentation of a Child Health History

Name: Sarah R.   Age: 32 months   Sex: female

Address: 214 Fifth Avenue   Telephone: 567-9931 (parent's home)

Date of Admission: December 1   Telephone: 572-9771 (father's workplace)

Medical Diagnosis: bilateral otitis media (BOM)   Allergies: None known

Source of History: mother (Michelle) and father (Jason)

Chief Complaints

"Pale for about 3 days. . . . not eating. . . . runny nose for a week. . . . cranky." Doctor says Sarah may have an "earache." Child crying on admission and saying "owie, owie."

Present Illness

Child has been sick for about 1 week. "Ran temperature for 2 days" and "had cough and runny nose. . . . Just didn't come around . . . didn't eat." Mother says she is really tired because she has been up with Sarah for about 3 nights. Worried about impact of BOM on Sarah's hearing; had niece who had a ruptured "eardrum" and had "speech problems." Dad feels mother may be "babying" Sarah because she spends so much time with Sarah.

Past Health History

Birth history

Patient delivered by normal, uncomplicated, vaginal delivery. Mom and Sarah in hospital for 2 days following delivery. No obvious congenital abnormalities detected at birth.

Feeding history

Child "slow to gain" as an infant. Weight at birth 3.4 kg. Weight at 1 year 7.8 kg. "Picky eater" and "had to have formula changed a lot" because of "gas and crying." Cereal introduced at 4 months, fruits at 6 months, vegetables at 7 months, and full diet with homogenized milk by 9 months, with no adverse effects. Now eats nearly everything except peas. Eats "a lot." Takes a chewable multivitamin daily. Weaned from bottle at 18 months.

Dietary recall

In the last 24 hours, child has had "about" 4 oz of milk, 8 oz of juice, bowl of soup, 2 crackers, an ice cream cone, and "2 spoonful" of rice.

Elimination history

"Constipated a lot when on formula . . . poops were hard and smelly." "Since going on homogenized milk has been better . . . still has hard stools if she drinks too much milk." Mom "limits" milk intake to about 16 oz a day and encourages child to drink juice. Child prefers juice to fruit or vegetables.

Childhood illnesses

Chickenpox at 1 year. Surgery for pyloric stenosis at 10 days.

Immunizations

2 mo—DTaP, IPV, Hib
4 mo—DTaP, IPV, Hib
6 mo—Hib   No untoward reactions
12 mo—IPV
15 mo—Hib, MMR
18 mo—DTaP, varicella

Current medications

Tylenol 80 mg (liquid) at 2 PM (2 hours ago) for fever.

Growth and Development History

General development

No delays noted on Denver II.

Physical growth

Weight pattern noted above. All "baby teeth" in by 21 months. Current weight 14.8 kg; height 51 cm. Completely toilet trained. Goes to bathroom on own; will ask to go "#1" or "#2."

Gross motor development

Rolled over from back to front and front to back by 5 months. Walked at 11 months. Able to jump with both feet and to stand on one foot momentarily.

Fine motor development

Holds crayon with fingers; able to copy circle; enjoys coloring.

Sleep

Child established uninterrupted nighttime sleep pattern at 6 months, but reverted to frequent night awakenings at 8 months. Mom says no changes in family or environment at this time. Since 8 months sleeps about 10 hours a night with frequent awakenings, which have no pattern. Child sometimes confused and crying when she awakens but at other times is calm. Mother responds to awakenings by taking child to bathroom and giving her a drink. If child does not immediately settle to crib after this, mom takes her into the family bed. Child does not have afternoon naps; goes down for night between 9 and 10 PM and gets up for day around 7:30 AM; generally is held and read to before bedtime; takes pink baby blanket to bed.

Language development

First word at 9 months. First phrases after 24 months. Vocalization on admission limited primarily to "owie" and crying; however, mom states that child is usually very talkative, easy to understand. Has trouble with "l's" and "y's"; for example, says "lellow" for yellow. Uses sentences of 4 or 5 words. "Gets upset if you don't understand her and sulks."

Social development

Recognizes familiar people, objects, and places. Initially shy with adults. Aggressive with other children; "bites and hits when she wants something." Parents use "time out" if child is aggressive or misbehaving. Dad feels spanking would be more effective; mom disagrees. Able to feed and dress self almost completely. "Very independent." "Occasional temper tantrums: screams and throws herself to ground . . . usually when meals are late." Has developed fear of "monsters."

Cognitive development

Alert; follows instructions to "sit up here" or "lie down."

Personal/Social History

Family has well-defined parameters. Parents see themselves as "separate" from their families and able to set own patterns of discipline. Michelle sees her mother's depression as sometimes troublesome and says her mother demands Michelle's time but has little time for her granddaughter. Jason and Michelle express conflict over discipline of Sarah. Both state that they have difficulty solving problems such as discipline because Jason "gets mad and walks out" and then Michelle withdraws for "awhile," which makes Jason mad. Family communication is "open" around matters involving household tasks and responsibilities but there is more difficulty with expressing emotion. Discipline of Sarah largely involves "time out." Father feels Sarah rules her mother sometimes, a perception not shared by Michelle. Couple states they have a wide network of friends, including Sarah's babysitter, to whom Sarah is "very attached." Michelle is a sales rep for a medical supply company; some college education. Jason is an engineer and has a university degree. See genogram and ecomap (see Figure E-1 on pages 356-357) for further information regarding internal and external family structures.

Systems Review

1. General

   Pale, tired-looking child; alert; clings to mother when first approached; moves without difficulty.
   Temperature: 38.2 (A)
   Pulse: 130 (apical)/min; regular
   Respiration: 30/min
   Blood pressure: 98/64
   Weight: 14.8 (clothed)
   Height: 51 cm (no shoes)

2. Integument

   Skin: Pale, warm; slightly dry in arm creases; elastic; no edema. Lesion approximately 2.5 cm in diameter, red, dry, and raised on left medial forearm "due to fall from tricycle 2 weeks ago." Indented area "old chickenpox scar" (approximately 2 mm) near left eyebrow.

Mucous membranes: Reddened, moist.

Nailbeds: Pink, texture firm, no clubbing; tooth imprints on left index finger "due to sucking."

Hair/scalp: Hair clean, soft, abundant on scalp. Scalp clean, no lesions.

3. Head and neck

Head: Normocephalic.

Neck: Full ROM, strong symmetrically; trachea at midline; thyroid not palpable. Firm, warm, diffuse nodes palpated in preauricular, submandibular, occipital, and cervical regions.

4. Ears

Auricle: No lesions, canals clean and free of cerumen.

Otoscopic examination: Drums bilaterally intact, red, and bulging; landmarks not present.

Hearing: Child asked for directions to be repeated on nearly every occasion. Rinne and Weber's tests; unable to gain child's cooperation sufficiently to gain accurate assessments.

5. Eyes

Vision: Able to name 4 of 7 cards on two tries at 4.6 m.

Extraocular movement: No deviation with cover test, light reflex equal. Unable to gain cooperation in fields of vision testing.

Conjunctiva: Clear.

Sclerae: Clear, white.

Iris: Blue, round.

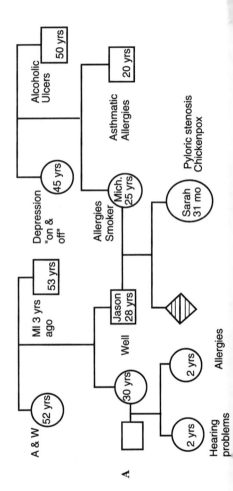

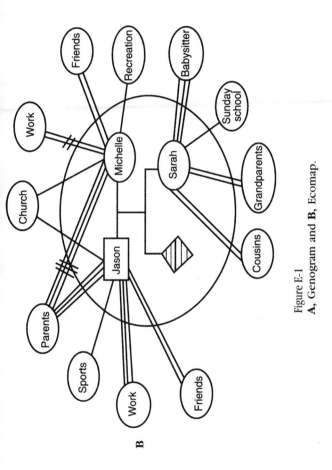

Figure E-1
A, Genogram and B, Ecomap.

Pupils: PERRLA.

Ophthalmoscopic examination: Disc round, creamy white; macular areas normal; normal veins and arteries.

Lacrimal system: No swelling, excess tearing.

Corneal reflex: Present.

6. Face, nose, and oral cavity

Face, nose, and facial movements: Symmetric; child solemn but smiles with encouragement; marked shadows under both eyes; external nares excoriated, green thick nasal discharge present; no pain on palpation of cheeks and areas above eyebrows; septum slightly deviated to left.

Oral cavity: Lips dry, pale, and slightly cracked; oral membranes moist, pink, no lesions.
Gums: No edema or swelling.
Teeth: Clean, all present. Both upper, central incisors protrude slightly.
Tonsils red and almost to uvula: adenoids visible; voice hoarse.

7. Thorax and lungs

Thorax slightly oval, symmetric at rest. No indrawings. Respirations diaphragmatic. Tactile fremitus equal bilaterally. Vesicular sounds heard through lung fields. No adventitious sounds.

8. Cardiovascular system

Heart: PMI in 4 ICS; no abnormal pulsations palpated, $S_1 > S_2$ in mitral, tricuspid areas and at Erb's point. Systolic murmur heard in third intracostal space.

Vascular system: Radial and peripheral pulses equal, regular, and strong.

9. Abdomen

   Healed scar in epigastric region (pyloric stenosis), abdomen protruberant, symmetric; no bulging, bowel sounds 4 to 5/min in each quadrant; firm mass palpated in lower left quadrant (last bowel movement 4 days ago), no hernias.

10. Genitourinary/reproductive system

    Breasts: Nipples symmetric, areola pink; no discharge.

    Genitalia: Labia approximate and are intact; vagina pink, no discharge.

11. Musculoskeletal system

    Muscular development and mass normal for age; movements symmetric; gait normal; feet slightly flattened; all digits present; joints nontender, not swollen; full range of motion; Kernig's sign negative.

12. Nervous system

    Mental status: Child follows directions appropriately when direction repeated.

    Cranial nerve function: Not done.

    Motor function: Muscle strength equal and symmetric.

Related Nursing Diagnoses

Anxiety: Related to hospitalization; pain.

Constipation: Related to decreased fluid and food intake; decreased mobility; and food preferences.

Communication, impaired verbal: Related to fear; anxiety; and decreased hearing abilities.

Family processes, alterations in: Related to child with infection; conflict between parents related to childrearing practices.

Fear: Related to hospitalization; fantasies.

Fluid volume deficit, potential: Related to reduced oral intake.

Knowledge deficit: Related to establishment of sleep patterns in toddlers; parenting practices.

Nutrition, altered: Less than body requirements related to loss of appetite.

Pain: Related to pressure caused by inflammatory process and discomfort in swallowing.

Parental role conflict: Related to dysfunctional communication and problem solving around discipline issues.

Sleep pattern disturbance: Related to fears; trained night crying; and/or pain.

Bibliography

Adler J: Patient assessment: abnormalities of the heartbeat, *Am J Nurs* 77:647-673, 1977.

All N, Siktberg L: Osteoporosis prevention in female adolescents: calcium intake and exercise participation, *Ped Nurs* 27:132, 135-138, 2001.

Ahmann E, Lawrence J: Exploring language about families, *Ped Nurs* 25:221-224, 1999.

American Academy of Pediatrics: *Report of the committee on infectious diseases,* Elk Grove, IL, 1991, The Academy.

Amoateng-Adjepong Y et al: Accuracy of an infrared tympanic thermometer, *Chest* 115:1002-1005, 1999.

Androkites AL et al: Comparison of axillary and infrared tympanic membrane thermometry in a pediatric oncology outpatient setting, *J Pediatr Oncol Nurs* 15:216-222, 1998.

Arvidson CR: The adolescent gynecologic exam, *Ped Nurs* 25:71-74, 1999.

Baker NC et al: The effect of thermometer and length of time inserted on oral temperature measurements of afebrile subjects, *Nurs Res* 33(2):109-111, 1984.

Ball J, Bindler R: *Pediatric nursing,* ed 2, Stamford, CT, 1999, Appleton & Lange.

Beckmann MR, Procter-Zentner J: *Nursing assessment and promotion: strategies across the lifespan,* Norwalk, CT, 1993, Appleton & Lange.

Beecroft PC, Redick S: Possible complications of intramuscular injections on the pediatric unit, *Ped Nurs* 15:333-336, 1989.

Bellman M, Kennedy N: *Pediatrics and child health,* London, 2000, Churchill Livingstone.

Berkey K, Hanson SM: *Pocket guide to family assessment and intervention,* St Louis, 1991, Mosby.

Bickley LS: *Bates' guide to physical examination and history taking,* ed 7, Philadelphia, 1999, JB Lippincott.

Boszormenyi-Nagy I, Spark G: *Invisible loyalties,* New York, 1984, Brunner/Mazel.

Brennan A: Caring for children during procedures: a review of the literature, *Ped Nurs* 20:451-457, 1994.

Bresnahan K et al: Prenatal cocaine use: impact on infants and mothers, *Ped Nurs* 17:123-129, 1991.

Broome ME: Preparation of children for painful procedures, *Ped Nurs* 16:490-496, 1990.

Brunner LS, Suddarth DS: *Lippincott manual of nursing practice,* Philadelphia, 1993, JB Lippincott.

Burten C, Metzger B: Childhood obesity and risk of cardiovascular disease: a review of the science, *Ped Nurs* 26:13-17, 2000.

Calamero CJ: Infant nutrition in the first year of life: tradition or science? *Ped Nurs* 26:211-215, 2000.

Chernecky C, Berger BJ: *Laboratory tests and diagnostic procedures,* ed 3, Philadelphia, 2001, WB Saunders.

Clark MC: In what ways, if any, are child abusers different from other parents? *Health Visit* 62:268-270, 1989.

Clark MJ: *Nursing in the community,* Stamford, CT, 1999, Appleton & Lange.

Clubb R: Chronic sorrow: adaptation patterns of parents with chronically ill children, *Ped Nurs* 17:461-465, 1991.

Cohen SM: Lead poisoning: a summary of treatment and prevention, *Ped Nurs* 27:125-127, 2001.

Cormier LS et al: *Interviewing helping skills for health professionals,* Monterey, CA, 1984, Wadsworth Health Sciences Division.

Danielson CB, Hamel-Bissel B, Winstead-Fry P: *Families, health, and illness, perspectives on coping and intervention,* St Louis, 1993, Mosby.

D'Apolito K: Substance abuse: infant and childhood outcomes, *Ped Nurs* 13:307-315, 1998.

De la Cuesta C: Relationships in health visiting: enabling and mediating, *Int J Nurs Stud* 31:451-459, 1994.

Doegnes M, Moorhouse M: *Nurse's pocket guide: nursing diagnoses with interventions,* ed 7, Philadelphia, 1998, FA Davis.

Downs MP, Sliver NK: The "A.B.C.D." to H.E.A.R.: early identification in nursery, office, and office of the infant who is deaf, *Clin Pediatr* 11:563-565, 1972.

Dunst C et al: *Enabling and empowering families,* Cambridge, MA, 1988, Brookline Books.

Edelstein S: Nutritional assessment in cancer cachexia, *Ped Nurs* 17: 237-240, 1991.

Engle MA: Heart sounds and murmurs in the diagnosis of heart disease, *Pediatr Ann* 10:18-31, March 1987.

Faux SA et al: Intensive interviewing with children and adolescents, *World J Nurs Rev* 10:180-194, 1988.

Frankenberg WK et al: The Denver II: a major revision and restandardization of the Denver Developmental Screening tool, *Pediatrics* 89:91-97, 1992.

Frohlich ED et al: Recommendations for human blood pressure determination by sphygmomanometers: report of special task force appointed by the steering committee, American Heart Association, *Circulation* 77:501A, 1988.

Gage RE: Consequences of children's exposure to spouse abuse, *Ped Nurs* 16:258-260, 1990.

Gordon M: *Manual of nursing diagnosis,* ed 9, St Louis, 2000, Mosby.

Gordon S: Lyme disease in children, *Ped Nurs* 20:415-418, 1994.

Gryskiewicz JM, Huseby TC: The pediatric abdominal assessment: a multiple challenge, *Postgrad Med* 67:126-128, 1980.

Hartley B, Fuller CC: Juvenile arthritis: a nursing perspective, *J Ped Nurs* 12:100-106, 1997.

Heiney SP: Helping children through painful procedures, *Am J Nurs* 91(11):20-24, 1991.

Hoeckelman RA et al: *Primary pediatric care,* ed 4, St Louis, 2001, Mosby.

Hoffman C et al: Evaluation of three brands of tympanic thermometers, *Can J Nurs Res* 31:117-131, 1999.

Hole JW: *Human anatomy and physiology,* ed 2, Dubuque, IA, 1981, William C. Brown.

Houck GM, King MC: Child maltreatment: family characteristics and developmental consequences, *Issues in Mental Health Nurs* 10:193-208, 1989.

Houlder LC: The accuracy and reliability of tympanic thermometry compared to rectal and axillary sites in young children, *Ped Nurs* 26:311-314, 2000.

Hunter LP: Measurement of axillary temperatures in neonates, *World J Nurs Rev* 13:324-335, 1991.

Jackson MM, McLeod RP: Tuberculosis in infants, children, and adolescents: an update with case studies, *Ped Nurs* 23:411-415, 1998.

Johnson BH: Children's drawings as a projective technique, *Ped Nurs* 16:11-17, 1990.

Johnson TS et al: Reliability of three measurement techniques in term infants, *Ped Nurs* 25:13-17, 1999.

Johnstone HA, Marcinak JF: Sibling abuse: another component of domestic violence, *J Ped Nurs* 12:51-53, 1997.

Josephs JE: Pertussis in the adolescent and adult: a primary care concern, *Clin Excellence Nurse Pract* 4:361-365, 2000.

Kahn-D'Angelo L: Serious head injury during the first year of life, *Phys Occup Ther Pediatr* 9(4):49-59, 1989.

Kaslow FW: *Voices in family psychiatry,* Newbury Park, CA, 1990, Sage.

Kelley SJ et al: Birth outcomes, health problems and neglect with prenatal exposure to cocaine, *Ped Nurs* 17:130-136, 1991.

Kim MJ et al: *Pocket guide to nursing diagnoses,* ed 7, St Louis, 1997, Mosby.

Kluger M: Fever, *Pediatrics* 66:720-723, 1980.

Knauth DG: Marital change during the transition to parenthood, *Ped Nurs* 27:169-172, 184, 2001.

Krowchuck H: Child abuser stereotypes: consensus among clinicians, *Appl Nurs Res* 2:35-39, 1989.

LaMontagne L: Bolstering personal control in child patients through coping interventions, *Ped Nurs* 19:235-237, 1993.

Lanham DM et al: Accuracy of tympanic temperature readings in children under 6 years of age, *Ped Nurs* 25:39-42, 1999.

Leahey M, Wright LM: *Families and life-threatening illness,* Springhouse, PA, 1987, Springhouse.

Lefrancois GR: *Of children,* Belfmont, CA, 1977, Wadsworth.

Lewin L: Establishing a therapeutic relationship with an abused child, *Ped Nurs* 16:263-264, 1990.

Liebermann A: *Community and home health nursing,* Springhouse, PA, 1990, Springhouse Corporation.

Loranger N: Play intervention strategies for the Hispanic toddler with separation anxiety, *Ped Nurs* 18:571-574, 1992.

Lynch M: Special children, special needs: the ectodermal dysplasias, *Ped Nurs* 18:212-216, 1992.

Manian FA, Griesenauer S: Lack of agreement between tympanic and oral measurement in adult hospitalized patients, *Am J Infect Control* 26:428-430, 1998.

Marino BL, Lipshitz M: Temperament in infants and toddlers with cardiac disease, *Ped Nurs* 17:445-448, 1991.

McFarlane J, Soeken K: Weight gain of infants, age birth to 12 months, born to abused women, *Ped Nurs* 25:19-22, 1999.

Meeropol E: Parental needs assessment: a design for nurse specialist practice, *Ped Nurs* 17:456-458, 1991.

Montville NH, White MA: Diagnosis and pharmacological management of acute otitis media, *Ped Nurs* 23:423-425, 1998.

Mosby's medical, nursing and allied health dictionary, ed 5, St Louis, 1998, Mosby.

Murry S et al: Screening families with young children for child maltreatment potential, *Ped Nurs* 26:47-51, 2000.

Muscari ME, Milks CJ: Assessing acute abdominal pain in females, *Ped Nurs* 21:215-220, 1995.

O'Brien E: Detection and removal of head lice with an electronic comb: zapping the louse! *J Ped Nurs* 13:265-266, 1998.

Pagana K, Pagana TJ: *Diagnostic testing and laboratory test reference,* ed 5, St Louis, 2001, Mosby.

Patrick ML et al: *Medical-surgical nursing,* Philadelphia, 1991, JB Lippincott.

Perry AG, Potter PA: *Clinical nursing skills and techniques,* ed 4, St Louis, 1998, Mosby.

Pillitteri A: *Child health nursing: care of the child and family,* Philadelphia, 1999, JB Lippincott.

Pillsbury D: *Manual of dermatology,* Philadelphia, 1971, WB Saunders.

Potter PA: *Pocket guide to health assessment,* ed 4, St Louis, 1998, Mosby.

Quick G, Sicilio M: When should you suspect child abuse? A photographic guide: part 1: cutaneous lesions, *Consultant* 29(7):31-39, 1989.

Quick G, Sicilio M: When should you suspect child abuse? A photographic guide: part 3: neurologic manifestations, *Consultant* 29(7): 70-76, 1989.

Ramirez M: *Psychotherapy and counseling with minorities: a cognitive approach to individual and cultural differences,* Toronto, 1991, Pergamon Press.

Report of the second task force on blood pressure control in children, 1987, *Pediatrics* 1-25, 1987.

Rice R: *Manual of home health nursing procedures,* ed 2, St Louis, 2000, Mosby.

Robertson J: Pediatric pain assessment: validation of a multidimensional tool, *Ped Nurs* 19:209-213, 1993.

Rogers J et al: Evaluation of use of tympanic membrane thermometer in pediatric patients, *Ped Nurs* 17:376-378, 1991.

Schroeder B, McEroy-Shields K: Visual acuity, binocular vision, and ocular muscle balance in WLBW children, *Ped Nurs* 17:30-33, 1991.

Schultz A et al: Preverbal, early verbal pediatric pain scale (PEPPS): development and early psychometric testing, *J Ped Nurs* 14:19-26, 1999.

Schuster C, Ashburn S: *The process of human development: a holistic lifespan approach,* Boston, 1986, Little, Brown.

Selikman J: The multiple focus of immune deficiency in children, *Ped Nurs* 16:351-355, 361, 1990.

Sganga A et al: A comparison of four methods of normal newborn temperature measurement, *Mater Child Nurs* 25:76-79, 2000.

Sherwen LN et al: *Maternity nursing: care of the childbearing family,* Stamford, CT, 1999, Appleton & Lange.

Silverman BG et al: The use of infrared ear thermometers in pediatric and family practice offices, *Public Health Rep* 113:268-272, 1998.

Smith J: Are electronic thermometry techniques suitable alternatives to traditional mercury thermometers in the pediatric setting? *J Adv Nurs* 28:1030-1039, 1998.

Spector RE: *Cultural diversity in health and illness,* Upper Saddle River, NJ, 2000, Prentice Hall.

Stanhope M, Knollmueller RN: *Handbook of community and home health nursing,* St Louis, 1992, Mosby.

Stanhope M, Lancaster J: *Community health nursing: Process and practice for promoting health,* St Louis, 1992, Mosby.

Stewart MJ: *Community nursing: promoting Canadians' health,* Toronto, 1995, WB Saunders.

Stuart G, Sundeen SJ: *Principles and practice of psychiatric nursing,* ed 6, St Louis, 1998, Mosby.

Stulginsky M: Nurses' home health experience: part II: the unique demands of home visits, *Nurs Health Care* 14:476-485, 1993.

Sutter K et al: Reliability of head circumference measurements in preterm infants, *Ped Nurs* 23:485-486, 1997.

Terkelson K: Toward a theory of family life cycle. In Carter EA, McGoldrick M, editors: *The famly life cycle: a framework for family therapy,* New York, 1980, Gardner.

Tessler MD et al: Pain behaviors: postsurgical responses of children and adolescents, *J Ped Nurs* 13:41-46, 1998.

Vessey J: Developmental approaches to examining young children, *Ped Nurs* 21:53-57, 1995.

Wadsworth BJ: *Piaget's theory of cognitive and affective development,* ed 4, New York, 1989, Longman.

Wallace C, Farrington E: Pediatric drug information, *Ped Nurs* 17: 372-374, 1991.

Washburn P: Identification, assessment, and referral of adolescent drug abusers, *Ped Nurs* 17:137-140, 1991.

Waxler-Morrison N, Anderson J, Richardson E: *Cross-cultural caring: a handbook for professionals in Western Canada,* Vancouver, 1990, UBC Press.

Weber J, Kelley J: *Health assessment in nursing,* Philadelphia, 1998, JB Lippincott.

Weiss ME et al: A comparison of temperature measurements using three ear thermometers, *Appl Nurs Res* 11:158-166, 1998.

Williams SR: *Nutrition and diet therapy,* ed 8, St Louis, 1998, Mosby.

Wilson CJ, Mason M: Preparation for routine physical examination, *Child Health Care* 19:178-182, 1990.

Wong DL, Perry SE, Hockenberry MJ: *Maternal child nursing care,* ed 2, St Louis, 2001, Mosby.

Wong DL et al: *Whaley & Wong's nursing care of infants and children,* ed 6, St Louis, 1999, Mosby.

Wright L, Leahey M: *Nurses and families: a guide to family assessment and intervention,* Philadelphia, 2000, FA Davis.

Index